Cognitive Behavioral Therapy - Theories and Applications

Edited by Sandro Misciagna

Published in London, United Kingdom

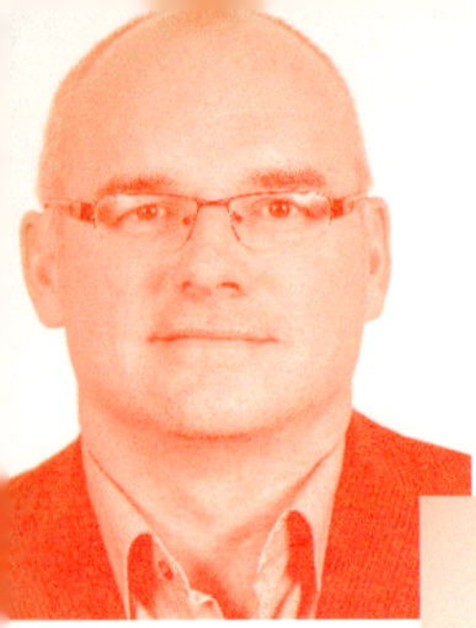
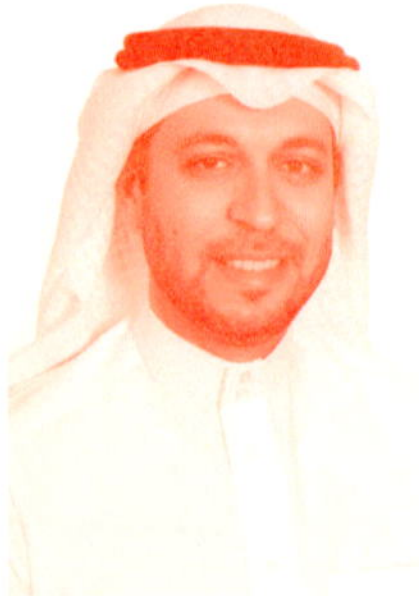
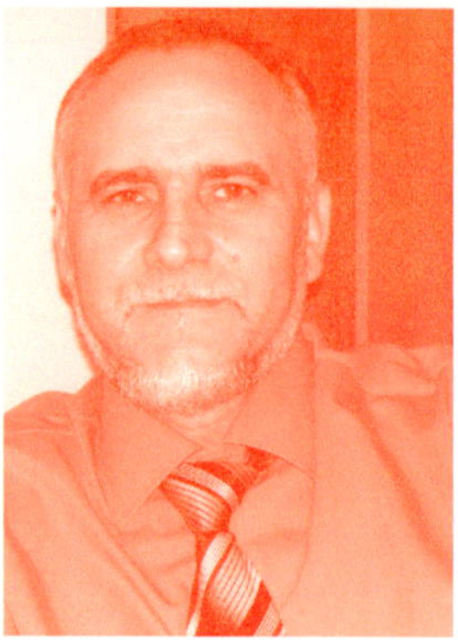
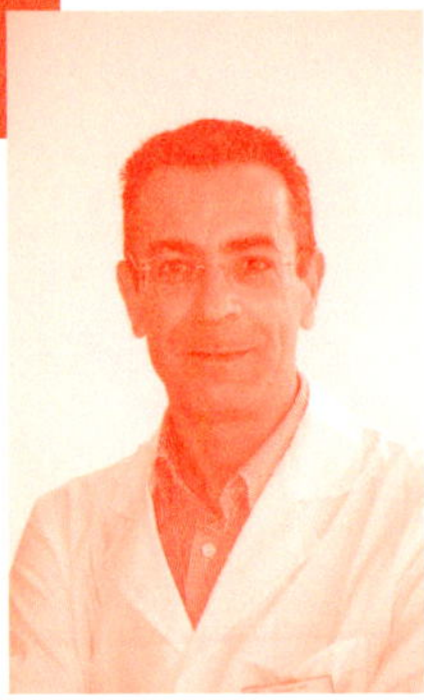
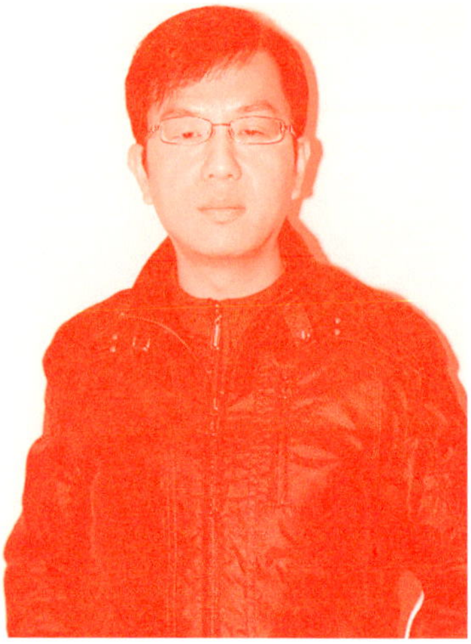
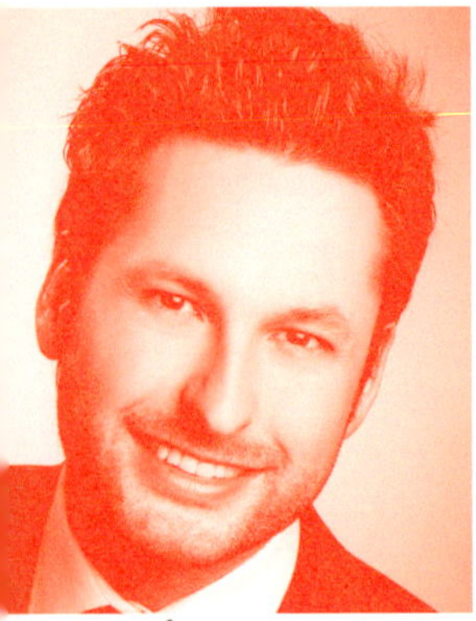
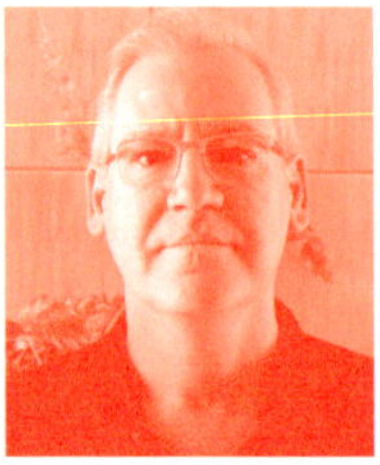

IntechOpen

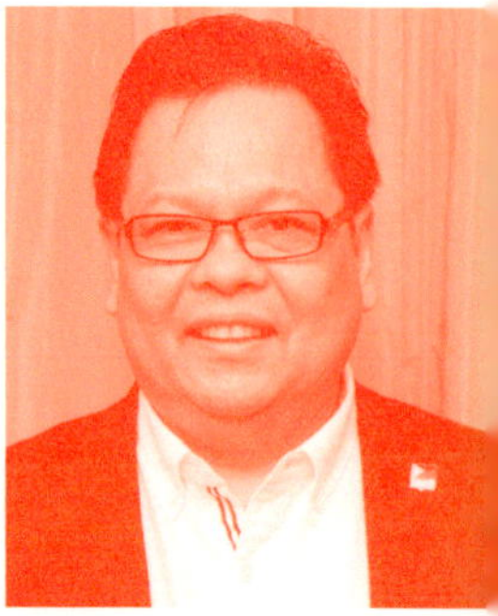
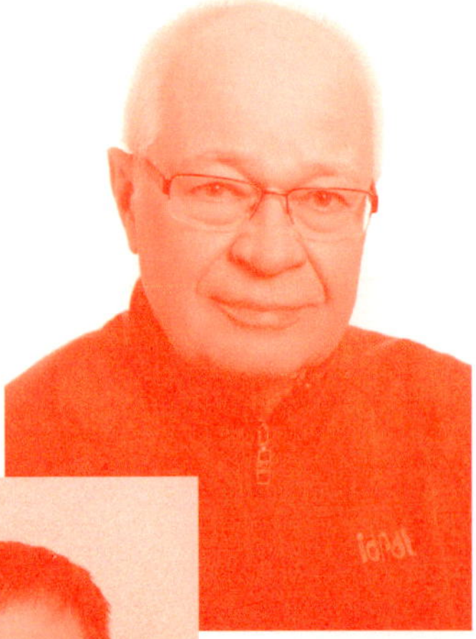
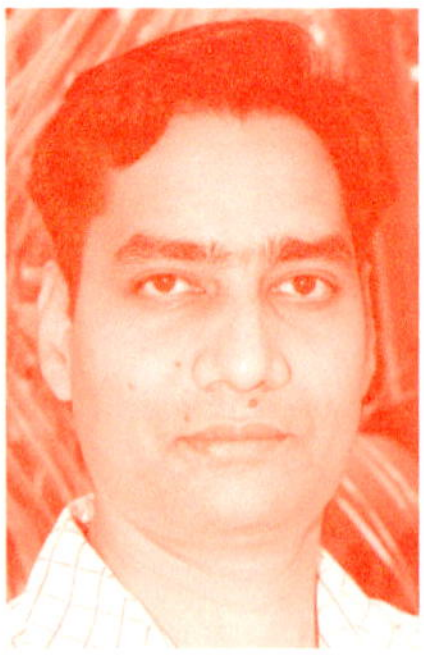
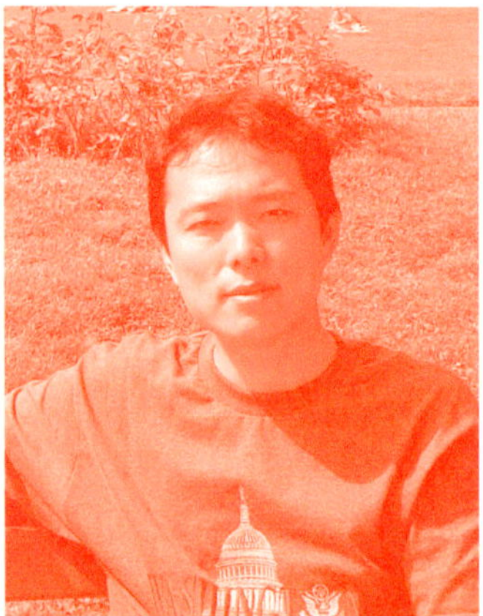
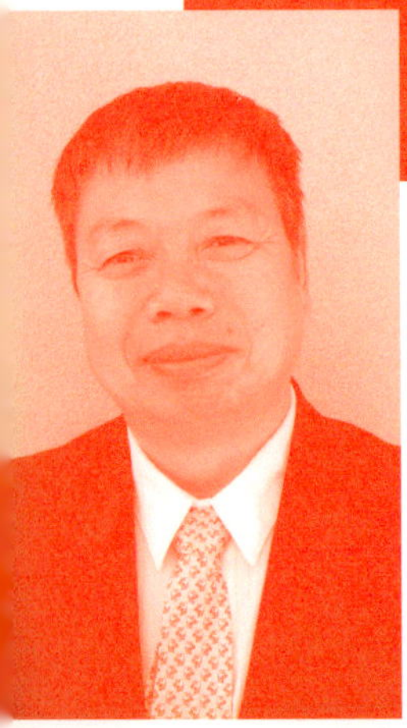
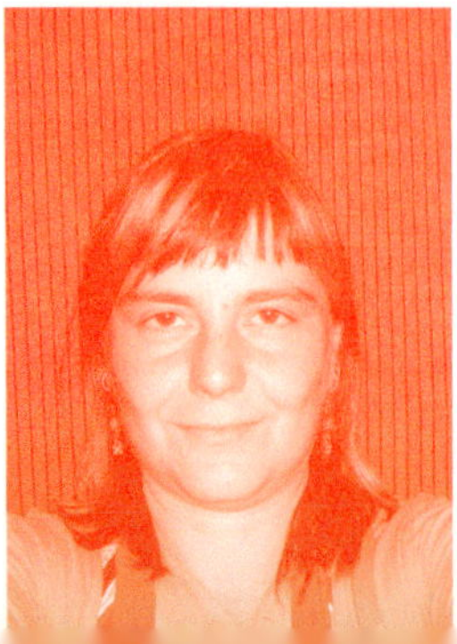

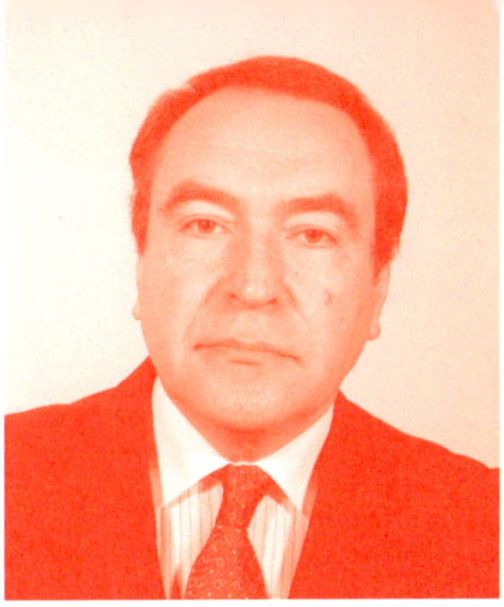

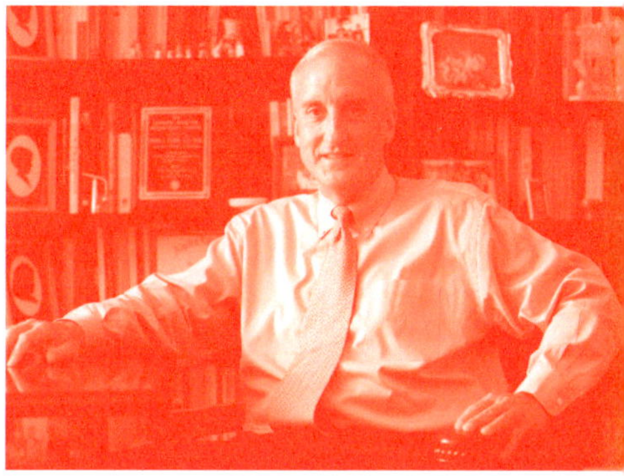

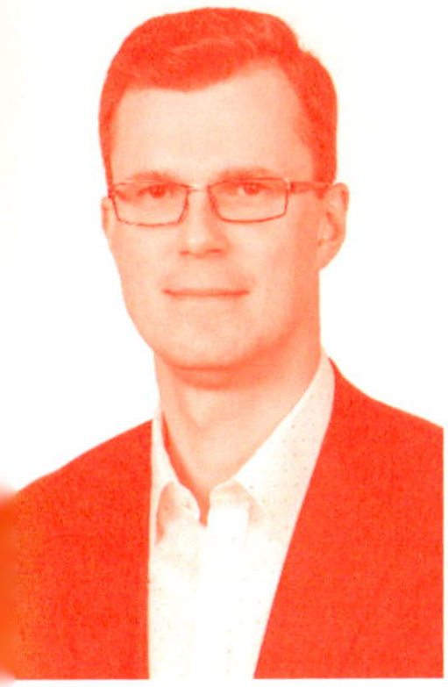

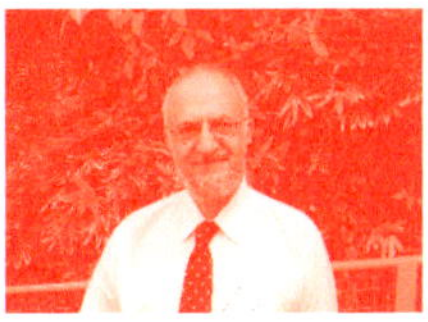

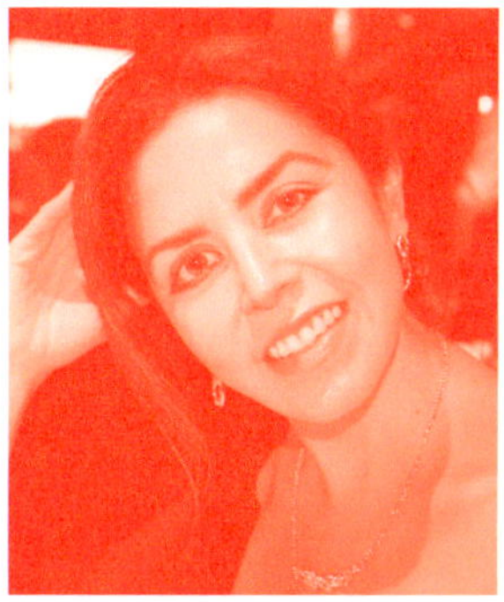

Supporting open minds since 2005

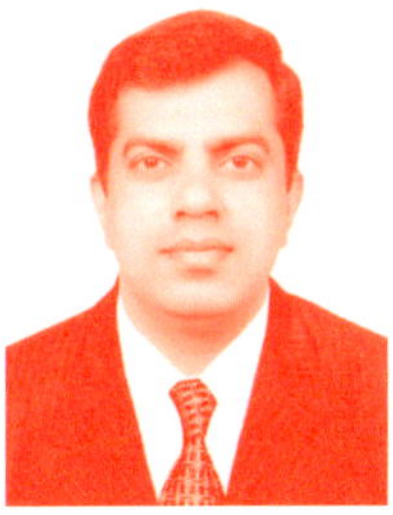

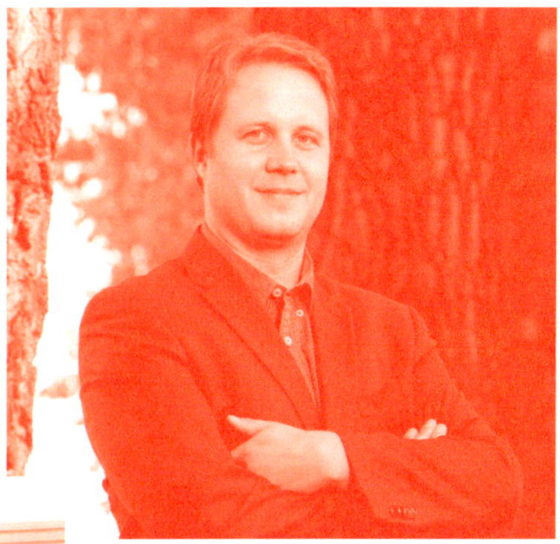

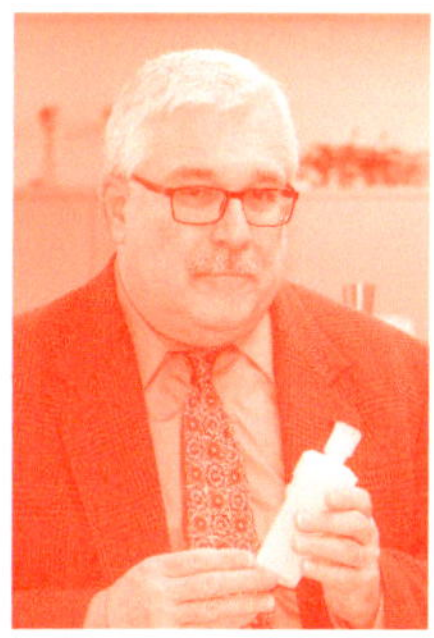

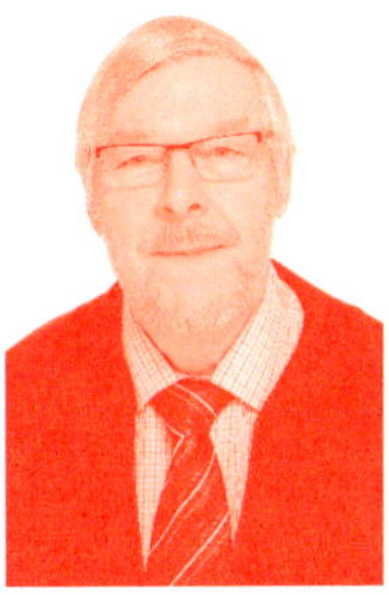

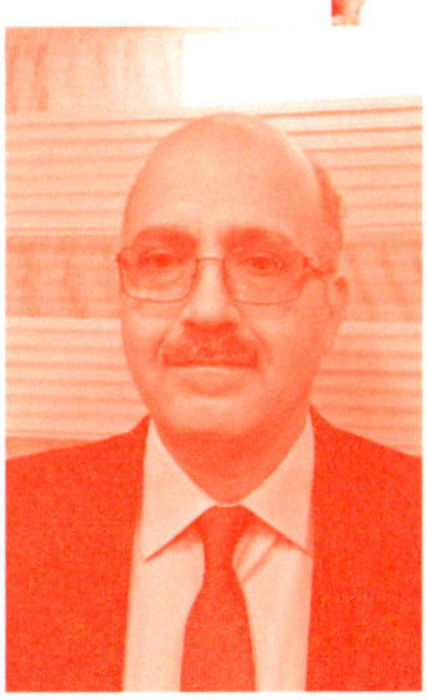

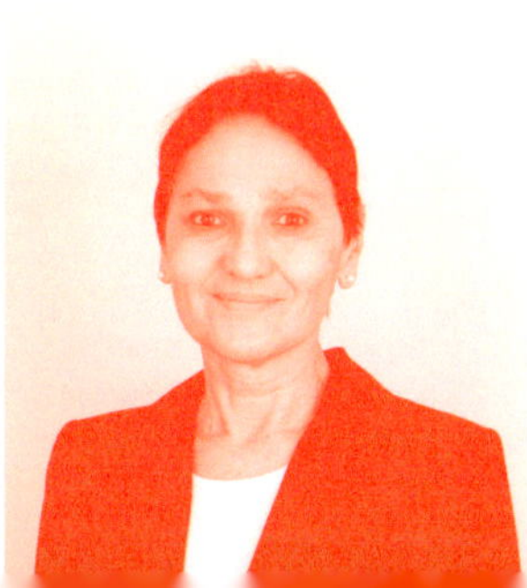

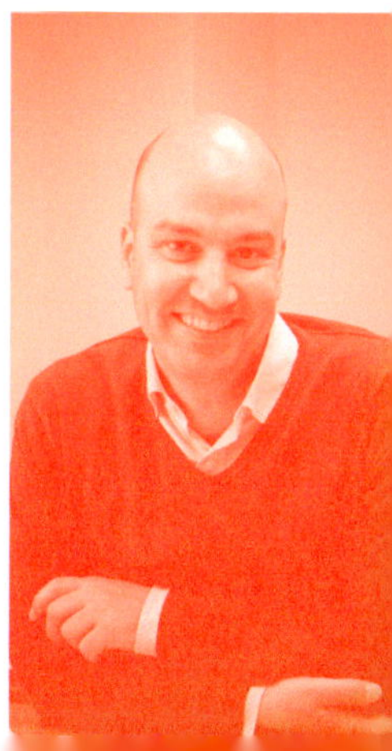

Cognitive Behavioral Therapy - Theories and Applications
http://dx.doi.org/10.5772/intechopen.78446
Edited by Sandro Misciagna

Contributors
Oleg Evgenevich Backsanskiy, Rosmawati Mohamad Rasit, Norzihan Ayub, Patricia Joseph Kimong, Guan Teik Ee, Michael L. Commons, Mansi Shah, Mark H. Keffer, Prisla Ücker Calvetti, Gabriel Gauer, Fernanda de Vargas, Sandro Misciagna, Siti Zuhrah Che Ab Razab

First published in London, United Kingdom, 2020 by IntechOpen
IntechOpen is the global imprint of INTECHOPEN LIMITED, registered in England and Wales, registration number: 11086078, 7th floor, 10 Lower Thames Street, London, EC3R 6AF, United Kingdom
Printed in Croatia

British Library Cataloguing-in-Publication Data
A catalogue record for this book is available from the British Library

Additional hard and PDF copies can be obtained from orders@intechopen.com

Cognitive Behavioral Therapy - Theories and Applications
Edited by Sandro Misciagna
p. cm.
Print ISBN 978-1-83962-165-9
Online ISBN 978-1-83962-164-2
eBook (PDF) ISBN 978-1-83962-163-5

For EU product safety concerns:
IN TECH d.o.o., Prolaz Marije Krucifikse Kozulić 3, 51000 Rijeka, Croatia, info@intechopen.com or visit our website at intechopen.com.

Meet the editor

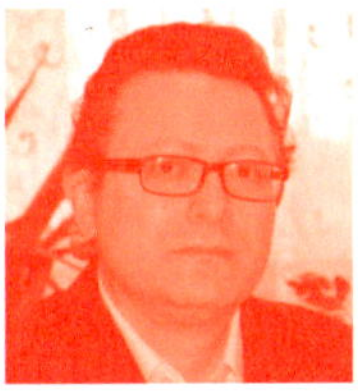

Dr. Sandro Misciagna was born on March 15, 1969 in Italy. He received his degree in medicine in 1995 and in neurology in 1999 at the Catholic University in Rome. From 1993 to 1995 he attended a research laboratory involved in cerebellar functions in mice. From 1994 to 2003 he attended the Neuropsychological Department of the Catholic University involved in human cognitive and behavioral disorders, writing various publications and book chapters. From 2001 to 2003 he was a teacher of clinical neuropsychology, clinical neurology, and cognitive rehabilitation mainly at the Catholic University. In 2003 he took a PhD in Neuroscience at the Catholic University discussing behavioral and cognitive profiles of patients with frontotemporal dementia. As a clinician he has worked in different neurological departments in Italian hospitals, Alzheimer's clinics, neuropsychiatric clinics, and neurological rehabilitative departments. From November 2016 he worked as a clinical neurologist in the Neurological Department and Stroke Unit of Belcolle Hospital in Viterbo. Recent interests include patients with epilepsy and epileptic seizure, neurophysiological studies, and antiepileptic pharmacological therapies.

Contents

Preface

Cognitive behavioral therapy (CBT) is a modern form of short-term psychotherapy based on the idea that the way an individual thinks and feels affects the way he or she behaves.

The core premise of this treatment approach was pioneered by Albert Ellis, who in 1957 introduced the name "rational emotive therapy" to emphasize its focus on emotional outcomes. Successively, Aaron Beck in 1976 created "cognitive therapy," which served as the basis for the development of CBT.

According to Beck's formulation, maladaptive cognitions, which consist of general beliefs or schemas about the self, the world, and the future, contribute to the maintenance of emotional distress and behavioral problems. According to this model, specific therapeutic strategies that change maladaptive cognitions lead to changed emotional distress and problematic behaviors.

In 1995, Ellis created the term "rational emotive behavior therapy" because behavioral factors constitute a fundamental component of this treatment approach. More recently, practitioners and scholars started to call it rational-emotive and "cognitive-behavior therapy" to emphasize its role in the CBT paradigm.

Since these early models, CBT has developed appropriate protocols to treat subjects of almost every age such as children, adolescents, adults, or the elderly and for individuals, families, and couples.

CBT integrates cognitive science and behavioral theories that are combined with clinical psychology and concludes that the way people perceive a situation determines their reaction more than the actual reality of the situation.

CBT provides useful tools that can be used to induce or facilitate belief revision such as cognitive restructuring or exposure/response prevention; these protocols have been applied both in groups and in individuals, even if the individual format is used more frequently than the group format.

This treatment plan uses patient collaboration as a motivating factor to generate changes in behavior, beliefs, and habits that can be self-reinforced. In fact, CBT gets patients actively involved in their treatment so that they understand that the way to improve their lives is to adjust their thinking and their approach to everyday situations.

The overall goal of this treatment is symptom reduction, improvement in functioning, and remission of the disorder.

CBT protocols are effective in the treatment of a vast variety of mental disorders, such as generalized anxiety disorders, somatoform disorders (such as hypochondriasis and body dysmorphic disorder), general stress or post-traumatic stress disorders, panic disorders (in particular with agoraphobia or social phobia), emotional disorders (depression, dysthymia), obsessive–compulsive disorders, problematic gambling, substance use disorder (such as nicotine, cannabis, opioid, or alcohol dependence), eating disorders (such as bulimia nervosa, binge-eating disorders), sleep dysfunction (especially insomnia), or to approach fatigue and chronic pain conditions, especially if associated with distress.

CBT is probably effective also for psychotic disorders especially on positive symptoms (i.e., delusions and/or hallucinations) of schizophrenia, personality disorders (including antisocial personality disorder), anger expression (anger, verbal and physical aggression, driving anger, anger suppression, and anger difficulties), and bipolar disorders. CBT is particularly promising for schizophrenia patients who suffer from acute episodes of psychosis rather than a more chronic condition.

Neurofunctional studies have demonstrated that CBT induces brain activation and functional changes in the amygdala, insula, and anterior corticolimbic brain circuits that control cognitive, motivational, and emotional aspects of physiology and behavior.

CBT should be used by health professionals with experience and training in cognitive and behavioral therapies, especially when used for the treatment of anxiety and mood disorders.

This book, written by authors with expertise in CBT, is useful for both clinicians and psychotherapists who want to understand modern cognitive psychology and develop specific personalized treatment plans of CBT.

The book is divided in two sections: theories of cognitive behavioral psychology and examples of applications of cognitive behavioral practice in different psychological situations.

The first section of the book consists of three chapters on cognitive psychology and prosocial behavior.

The first chapter is an introductory chapter titled Introductory Chapter: Definition of Cognitive Behavioral Therapy and Its Principal Applications.

In the next chapter on cognitive psychology and modern education, Prof. Oleg Backsanskig discusses the role of the cognitive approach in modern society and in the modern era of computer digitalization. According to Prof. Backsanskig cognitive approaches influence human activity not only in scientific fields, but also in social, political, and economic interactions.

Backsanskig discusses the bases of multidisciplinary approaches to persons and society problems according to information theory that also supposes pragmatic knowledge. He discusses various cognitive approaches based on entropy or combinational theories.

The author, relying on the etymology of different words from past Greek and Latin philosophers but also modern philosophers, explains a modern view of perception that closely agrees with informational theory.

The third chapter is centered on the role of self-efficacy in forming prosocial behavior.

According to Dr. Rosmawati Mohamad Rasit, prosocial behavior consists of positive actions commonly practiced in socio-surroundings such as the action of helping, loving, and developing empathy with each other. The formation of prosocial behavior has a connection with one's self-efficacy that is a trait where one can make a sound judgment about his or her own decisions, so that they can achieve personal success.

The author describes the characteristics that are important in determining prosocial behavior, such as personality traits or religious values since it encourages its society to practice tolerance and kindness to others.

Psychological interventions influence positive social behavior; for example, investigations of social support and negative social exchange as studied by Eidelman and others.

Mohamad Rasit discusses the possibility that having data on negative social exchanges at the start of treatment may benefit the outcome of ideographic, case formulation-based, and cognitive behavioral therapy.

The second section of the book consists of three chapters that contain examples of psychological applications of cognitive behavioral practice.

The chapter by Dr. Norzihan Ayub et al. concerns CBT for body dysmorphic disorder that is a mental disorder associated with psychological symptoms such as preoccupations with defects in physical appearance that are not observable to others, repetitive behaviors in response to appearance concerns, preoccupations causing clinically significant distress or impairment in social areas of functioning, and preoccupations with body fat or weight, whose symptoms meet diagnostic criteria for eating disorders and other features such as avoidance behaviors, delusional beliefs, and skin picking.

In this chapter the authors discuss the clinical diagnosis of body dysmorphic disorder, similarities with other mental illnesses, clinical assessment, the serotonin or other neurotransmitter hypothesis to explain the onset of body distorted image. Finally, the authors discuss psychological interventions or techniques of CBT (such as psychoeducation, exposure, ritual prevention, perceptual retraining) needed to treat individuals with body dysmorphic disorder to contrast their negative perception on physical appearance, mentioning practical examples of the techniques of CBT.

In the chapter by Dr. Michael Lamport Commons et al. we have an example of the application of CBT in depressive disorders.

As the authors explain, the background and nature of existential crises are important since if unresolved they can cause depression.

The authors describe the questionnaire "Existential Crisis Instrument" created to assess and measure the severity of existential crisis on the bases of a study on 50 participants who had to answer questions about the meaning of life, philosophy of living, and relations with others.

The authors describe five existential crises on the basis of accessibility to choose: the early teenage crisis (in the phase of transition toward independence from family), the sophomore crisis (related to questions such as: Who am I? Who can I be?), the adult crisis (which concerns questions of increased complexity such as choice of religion, political party, familial dedication, level of attachment to others, etc.), the midlife crisis (which regards changes in personal goals, lifestyle, social roles, etc.), and the later-life crisis (usually triggered by retirement, losing a job, illness, or death of a loved one).

The study of existential crisis is important to begin an accurate and correct CBT, which can help to treat depression, recognizing negative patterns of thought and replacing them with healthier ways of thinking.

On this basis, CBT can be used to concentrate attention on the immediate present, focus on specific problems, take an educational approach, attribute to patients an active role in their learning using homework assignments, and develop multiple strategies such as role playing, imaging, guided discovery, and behavioral experiments.

The last chapter by Prof. Prisla Calvetti et al. is about neurosciences and emotional regulation, and can be considered an introduction to the development of cognitive behavioral techniques for psychiatric disorders such as aggression, bipolar disorders, or criminal behavior.

In this chapter the authors describe factors to be considered in structuring personality and behavioral control from adolescence to adult age.

These factors make evident the importance not only of biological factors such as genetic components or cerebral connections, but also the result of complex interactions with the environment to determine predisposition of psychological tracts and cognitive functions.

From a cognitive point of view, the authors emphasize the importance of dysfunction in executive functions, which can be studied using neuropsychological tasks based on go-no go modality.

Executive dysfunctions or dysexecutive syndromes are a warning of an alteration in the prefrontal cortex of the frontal lobe, which are areas related to impulsive control and can be used to understand predisposition to develop psychiatric disorders with regard to particular controls of impulses such as aggression or control of behavior as in antisocial personality disorders on the basis of criminal acts.

In their opinion it is important to evaluate elements such as repentance, empathy, commotion, motivation, chronicity, and severity of antisocial behavior to determine the modality of cognitive behavioral strategies in treating both hospitalized and non-hospitalized psychiatric patients.

In conclusion I hope that this book can be useful to better understand CBT techniques used for a wide range of psychological problems or to develop specific CBT protocols since there is a clear need for high-quality studies examining the efficacy of CBT especially when compared with other psychological interventions, specific behavioral interventions, psychoeducational approaches, counseling interventions, or pharmacotherapy.

Finally, I think we need more psychometrical instruments to measure the CBT mechanism of change, and systematic studies to analyze the mechanism of cerebral functional changes induced by cognitive behavioral paradigms.

Sandro Misciagna, MD and PhD
Neurology Department and Stroke Unit,
Belcolle Hospital,
Viterbo, Italy

Section 1

Theories of Cognitive Behavioral Psychology

Chapter 1

Introductory Chapter: Definition of Cognitive Behavioral Therapy and Its Principal Applications

Sandro Misciagna

1. Story of modern cognitive behavioral therapy

Cognitive behavioral therapy (CBT) is a modern form of short-term psychotherapy based on the idea that the way an individual thinks and feels affects the way he behaves.

The core premise of this treatment approach was pioneered by Albert Ellis who in 1957 introduced the term "rational emotive therapy" (RET) to emphasize its focus on emotional outcomes. Successively, Aaron Beck in 1976 created "cognitive therapy" (CT), which served as the bases for the development of CBT.

According to Beck's formulation, maladaptive cognitions, which consist in general beliefs or schemas about the self, the world and the future, contribute to the maintenance of emotional distress and behavioral problems. According to this model, specific therapeutic strategies that change maladaptive cognitions lead to change emotional distress and problematic behaviors.

In 1995, Ellis created the term "rational emotive behaviour therapy" (REBT) because behavioral factors constitute a fundamental component of this treatment approach [1].

More recently, practitioners and scholars started to call it rational emotive and "cognitive behaviour therapy" to emphasize its role in CBT paradigm.

REBT protocols were applied in domains of clinical psychology, rational emotive education, organizational setting or counseling [2].

Since the late 1980s and 1990s, REBT was investigated in a series of randomized control trials that demonstrated its efficacy in many psychological conditions such as social phobia [3], obsessive–compulsive disorders [4], depression [5], psychotic symptoms [6] and behavioral disorders.

In 2013, on the bases of meta-analysis studies, REBT was included in the category of CBT [7] since its protocols are similar in structure with CBT protocols, while the main difference is that REBT specifically focuses on evaluative beliefs and not descriptive or inferential ones [8].

Since these early models, CBT have developed appropriate protocols to treat subjects of almost every age such as children, adolescent, adults or elderly and for individual, families and couples.

2. Principal applications of CBT

Cognitive behavioral therapy is an empirical and evidence-based psychotherapy that integrates cognitive science and behavioral theories, combined with clinical

IntechOpen

psychology, to conclude that the way people perceive a situation determines their reaction more than the actual reality of the situation does [9].

CBT provides useful tools that can be used to induce or facilitate belief revision such as cognitive restructuring or exposure/response prevention; these protocols have been applied both in groups and in individuals, even if the individual format is used more frequently than the group format.

This treatment plan uses patients' collaboration as a motivating factor, in order to generate changes in their behaviour, beliefs and habits that can be self-reinforced. In fact, CBT gets patients actively involved in their treatment so that they understand that the way to improve their lives is to adjust their thinking and their approach to everyday situations.

The overall goal of this treatment is symptom reduction, improvement in functioning and remission of the disorder. The initial sessions of CBT illustrate the close relationship between cognition and emotions. Each typical therapy session begins establishing an agenda of current problems, followed by cognitive restructuring of maladaptive cognitions. At the end of the session, the therapist assigns homework to help the patient to apply specific skills in his real life. Every step of CBT is reasoned and transparent. If the patient suffers from psychomotor retardation, behavioral strategies are implemented with cognitive interventions. The therapist can also use a series of questions to help the patients evaluate the utility and validity of their cognitions [10].

CBT consists in different protocols that are effective in the treatment of a vast variety of mental disorders, such as generalized anxiety disorders, panic disorders (in particular with agoraphobia or social phobia) and obsessive–compulsive disorders [11].

The session content varies for each specific disorder based on the empirically proven cognitive and behavioral model of each disorder. For example, cognitive themes concern about consequences of a panic attack (in phobia disorders), concern about social embarrassment (in social anxiety disorders), concern about dangers of worrying (in generalized anxiety disorders) and concern about consequences of intrusive thoughts (in obsessive–compulsive disorders).

CBT can be used to treat mood and emotional disorders such as depression or dysthymia [12]. With depressive disorders, the general therapeutic process of CBT is to split up into different steps, with an insistence on distinct therapeutic mechanisms, establishing a therapeutic relationship and managing maladaptive behaviors and cognitions.

CBT has been extensively tested for a wide range of neurotic and stress-related disorders such as general stress, post-traumatic stress disorders and somatoform disorders (such as hypochondriasis and body dysmorphic disorder) or medical problems with psychological components.

Several studies have demonstrated CBT utility in problematic gambling, substance use disorder (as nicotine, cannabis, opioid or alcohol dependence), eating disorders (as bulimia nervosa, binge eating disorders) [13] and sleep dysfunction (in particular insomnia) [14] or to approach fatigue, chronic pain conditions [15, 16] and inflammation pathologies [17], especially if associated with distress [18].

CBT is probably effective also for psychotic disorders associated with positive symptoms (i.e. delusions and/or hallucinations) in schizophrenia, personality disorders (including antisocial personality disorder) [19], anger expression (anger, verbal and physical aggression, driving anger, anger suppression and anger difficulties) and bipolar disorders. CBT is particularly promising for schizophrenia in patients who suffer from acute episode of psychosis rather than a more chronic condition [20].

Neurofunctional studies have demonstrated that CBT induces brain activation and functional changes in the amygdala, insula and anterior corticolimbic brain circuits that control cognitive, motivational and emotional aspects of physiology and behaviour [21].

CBT should be used by a health professional with experience and training in cognitive and behavioral therapies, especially when used for the treatment of anxiety and mood disorders.

This book, written by authors that are expertice in CBT, is useful both for clinicians and psychotherapists who wants to understand modern cognitive psychology and develop specific personalized treatment plans of cognitive behavioral therapy.

Author details

Sandro Misciagna
Neurology Department and Stroke Unit, Belcolle Hospital, Viterbo, Italy

*Address all correspondence to: sandromisciagna@yahoo.it

References

[1] Ellis A. Changing rational-emotive therapy (RET) to rational emotive behavior therapy (REBT). Journal of Rational-Emotive & Cognitive-Behavior Therapy. 1995;**13**(2):85-89

[2] David D. Rational Emotive Behavior Therapy. New York: Oxford University Press; 2014

[3] Mersch PPA, Emmelkamp PM, Bögels SM, Van der Sleen J. Social phobia: Individual response patterns and the effects of behavioral and cognitive interventions. Behaviour Research and Therapy. 1989;**27**(4):421-434

[4] Emmelkamp PM, Beens H. Cognitive therapy with obsessive-compulsive disorder: A comparative evaluation. Behaviour Research and Therapy. 1991;**29**(3):293-300

[5] David D, Szentagotai A, Lupu V, Cosman D. Rational emotive behavior therapy, cognitive therapy, and medication in the treatment of major depressive disorder: A randomized clinical trial, posttreatment outcomes, and six-month followup. Journal of Clinical Psychology. 2008;**64**(6):728-746

[6] Meaden A, Keen N, Aston R, Barton K, Bucci S. Cognitive Therapy for Command Hallucinations: An Advanced Practical Companion. New York: Routledge; 2013

[7] Cuijpers P, Berking M, Andersson G, Quigley L, Kleiboer A, Dobson KS. A meta-analysis of cognitive behavioural therapy for adult depression, alone and in comparison with other treatments. Canadian Journal of Psychiatry. 2013;**58**(7):376-385

[8] David D, Lynn SJ, Ellis A. Rational and Irrational Beliefs: Research, Theory, and Clinical Practice. Oxford: Oxford University Press; 2010

[9] Butler AC, Chapman JE, Forman EM, Beck AT. The empirical status of cognitive-behavioral therapy: A review of meta-analyses. Clinical Psychology Review. 2006;**26**:17-31

[10] Tarrier N, editor. Case Formulation in Cognitive Behaviour Therapy: The Treatment of Challenging and Complex Cases. New York: Routledge/Taylor & Francis Group; 2006

[11] Clark DM, Ehlers A, Hackmann A, et al. Cognitive therapy versus exposure and applied relaxation in social phobia: A randomized controlled trial. Journal of Consulting and Clinical Psychology. 2006;**74**:568-578

[12] Stubbings DR, Rees CS, Roberts LD, Kane RT. Comparing in-person to videoconference-based cognitive behavioral therapy for mood and anxiety disorders: Randomized controlled trial. Journal of Medical Internet Research. 2013;**15**(11):e258

[13] Valenzuela F, Lock J, Le Grange D, Bohon C. Comorbid depressive symptoms and self-esteem improve after either cognitive-behavioural therapy or family-based treatment for adolescent bulimia nervosa. European Eating Disorders Review. 2018;**26**(3):253-258. DOI: 10.1002/erv.2582. Epub: February 15, 2018

[14] Cheong MJ, Lee GE, Kang HW, Kim S, Kim HK, Jo HI, et al. Clinical effects of mindfulness meditation and cognitive behavioral therapy standardized for insomnia: A protocol for a systematic review and meta-analysis. Medicine (Baltimore). 2018;**97**(51):1-7

[15] Bach E, Beissner K, Murtaugh C, Trachtenberg M, Reid MC. Implementing a cognitive-behavioral pain self-management program in home health care. Part 2: Feasibility

and acceptability cohort study. Journal of Geriatric Physical Therapy (2001). 2013;**36**(3):130-137

[16] Beissner K, Bach E, Murtaugh C, Parker SJ, Trachtenberg M, Reid MC. Implementing a cognitive-behavioral pain self-management program in home health care. Part 1: Program adaptation. Journal of Geriatric Physical Therapy (2001). 2013;**36**(3):123-129

[17] Lopresti AL. Cognitive behaviour therapy and inflammation: A systematic review of its relationship and the potential implications for the treatment of depression. The Australian and New Zealand Journal of Psychiatry. 2017;**51**(6):565-582

[18] Hofmann S, Reinecke M, editors. Cognitive-Behavioral Therapy with Adults: A Guide to Empirically Informed Assessment and Intervention. Cambridge, UK: Cambridge University Press; 2010

[19] Sanatinia R, Wang D, Tyrer P, Tyrer H, Crawford M, Cooper S, et al. Impact of personality status on the outcomes and cost of cognitive-behavioural therapy for health anxiety. The British Journal of Psychiatry. 2016;**209**(3):244-250. DOI: 10.1192/bjp.bp.115.173526. Epub: July 21, 2016

[20] Morrison AP, Law H, Carter L, Sellers R, Emsley R, Pyle M, et al. Antipsychotic drugs versus cognitive behavioural therapy versus a combination of both in people with psychosis: A randomised controlled pilot and feasibility study. Lancet Psychiatry. 2018;**5**:411-423

[21] Lueken U, Straube B, Konrad C, Wittchen HU, Ströhle A, Wittmann A, et al. Neural substrates of treatment response to cognitive-behavioral therapy in panic disorder with agoraphobia. The American Journal of Psychiatry. 2013;**170**(11):1345-1355

Chapter 2

Cognitive Psychology and Modern Education

Oleg Evgenevich Baksansky

Abstract

The outlook of each certain person and society in general arises as result of mastering by them information on essence of the world and the nature of their interaction. Today, the methodological field of education is characterized by fragmentary vision, the complete picture of problems and uniform tradition of their statement, and interpretations that have not developed.

Keywords: education, cognitive science, education philosophy

1. Introduction to cognitive psychology

The swift development of information and communication technologies (ICTs) not only has qualitatively facilitated and accelerated an access to information but also led to an unprecedented synformism—the synthesis of information (databases) intrinsic to different scientific and technical fields. A formal (and external) unification is caused by the ICT foundation, computer digitization, indifferent to the object content, semantics. In a wonderful manner, a general digitization sends us back to a Hellenistic idea, natural numbers underlie the universe, which was suggested by Aristotle in *Metaphysics* in the discussion of Pythagorean propositions: "Everything in the nature is undoubtedly similar to numbers" and numbers are first in nature...and the elements of numbers are the elements of everything, and the whole heaven is harmony and number ([1], vol. 1, pp. 75–76).

However, such synthesis does not play a major role. In spite of subjective opinions and interests, the real paradigm—purposeful human activity—combines most different types of matter and interaction, such as natural, physicotechnological and scientific, social political, economical, international, military, and cultural.

2. Pragmatic approach to cognitive psychology

People and nature are inseparable worlds, and their intertwining becomes more tight with progress in science, technology, and civilization as a whole (e.g., it is quite reasonable to investigate military political problems in the context of geopolitical analysis). People make decisions and take actions according to strategic and tactical plans, which can be adequate and correct only if all significant factors and all participating persons are taken into account. Hence, when the problems of real pragmatics are analyzed, we deal, strictly speaking, with the system analysis of subjective and objective problems instead of recognizing a human role in the surrounding world.

In this approach, pragmatic problems are objectified to a great extent and can be regarded as the humanitarian and natural scientific problems of system analysis applied to pragmatic informational interactions: the decision-making based on analyzed pragmatic data and strategic planning. The essence of pragmatic research and theory is determined by (i) the completeness and quality of information and (ii) the validity, adequacy, and corroboration of pragmatic theories.

3. Cognitive approach of information theory

The information theory involves the multidisciplinary approaches to information problems and technologies ([2], p. 1). In addition, the informational interaction of entities of different kind is assumed to be the subject of new science synthesizing the results of natural sciences and humanities. In this chapter, pragmatic information and the foundations of pragmatic knowledge are analyzed. The architectonics of pragmatic theories is the subject of separate research.

Information appeared at the very beginning and contains the sources of plans and human actions. In the information theory, information of different type is understood as an intuitive description of objects and phenomena (in detail, ([2], p. 2)). According to the information theory, pragmatic information (from Greek πργματοζ signifying “action” or “manner”), that is, data on the real pragmatics, constitutes an information base according to which society objects make decisions, act, and create strategic plans ([2], p. 2). The pragmatics must start with a reliable information base if we want to engage in the real pragmatics instead of mythmaking.

The physical world, nature, can exist and exists as a whole, irrespectively of a person (as a carrier of activity, consciousness, and awareness ([3], p. 155)) and individual’s consciousness. In this sense, the physical world and its constituents are objective. Their fundamental property is that they can be observed and measured by both scientific instruments and a man. Facts—accurate results of observations and measurements—are empirical data. Natural scientific empirism allows *multiplication* (empirical repetition of a spontaneous observation and experiment), which helps to extract meaningful factors, filter a subjective component, formalize idealized speculative experiments, and define and verify initial hypotheses.

Observation and measurement tools must be available to any observer or researcher concerned to check factors. As was suggested by Vollmer [4], this requirement is is called intersubjective checkability. In addition, description tools must be intelligible (“intersubjective intelligibility”). In this case, Vollmer’s requirement of common language is optional because the translation requirement (the existence of faithful translation) is sufficient. Vollmer classifies these requirements (they are actually the condition of universalism) as “objectivity criteria.” Together with other criteria, they have been discussed in Kuznetsov et al. [5]. Comprehensively investigating the biological problems of a knowledge process and its expression tools (first of all, language), Maturana and Varela [6] also rely on the requirement that the phenomenon description (translation) intelligibility is a necessary condition of knowledge.

The foundation of perception and cognition is biological (the subject of investigation of the “evolutionary theory of knowledge”) [4, 6, 7]. In observation and perception of the real world (i.e., its physical and humanitarian aspects), the human physiological system is the same real tool as the physical world and the man-made technological facilities. The person-object coupling is described perfectly well in the striking metaphor of Lorenz [7], p. 260:

"Even in our days, a realist looks only at the external world and does not realize that he is its mirror. Even in our days, an idealist looks only at a mirror, averting his eyes from the external world. The direction of observation impedes them to see that the mirror has a nonreflective reverse side, relating it to the reflected real things: the physiological tool, the function of which is the cognition of the external world, has the same reality as this world."

4. Modern approach to cognitive psychology

In the light of the twentieth century discoveries in physics, an object and a subject (reference frame) are related more tightly than commonly thought: the object-perception dependence is also the immanent property of the physical world. The relativism noted by Lorenz is valid for physical objects proper: the fundamental attributes of bodies are noninvariant with respect to the reference frame. The most known attributes are size and shape (the abbreviation introduced by Lorenz) and time and age ("the clock paradox"). Together with physical laws, they can be noninvariant in different reference frames. This problem can be solved with the help of the "own reference frame" in which an object remains motionless. However, in the complicated system whose components move with respect to each other, the solution cannot be found. Thus, the Vollmer's "reality postulate" (discussed in Kuznetsov et al. [5]), that is, "there is the real world independent of perception," cannot be accepted.

5. Cognitive approaches based on entropy, algorithms and combinatorial theory

A quantitative description of information is usually associated with three approaches based on entropy [8], algorithms (Kolmogorov), and the combinatorial theory [2]. An advantage of these approaches is that they are supported by the developed mathematical apparatus. A disadvantage is that quantitative description makes it impossible to estimate the informational semantics—the meaningful content of information. A semantic approach was reported in the well-known study of Barr Hillel and Carnap [9] and developed by the author of Moscow semantic school, the foundations of which were provided by I.A. Vel'chuk and Y.A. Apresyan.

It is needless to say that the contents of many objects and processes of natural science have been described quantitatively (as functions, matrices, and equations).

The major part of information on the nature allows *multiplication*—accumulation in quantity (repetition of experiments). As a consequence of this fundamental property, natural scientific data can be checked and accepted by any researcher.

In contrary to objective information on the physical world, the basic part of pragmatic data is subjective. In essence, they are evidences, and not facts. Hence, the probability of distortion in an actual pattern is very high. For comprehensible reason, a general pattern contains information of different observers. Hence, distortions are added with contradictions. Data on a historical process can be assumed to be pragmatic.

Firstly, pragmatic data consist of evidences formed due to observations of experts and, hence, having the highest confidence. However, random and unintentional distortions must be taken into account. Secondly, they involve evidences of accidental persons, which are appreciably less reliable. It is obvious that the results of personal observations cannot be regarded as reliable. Thirdly, (this refers to the modern world), pragmatic data contain information recorded by observing devices or the governmental means of observation and inspection.

The events under consideration must be supplemented with man-made things and those not made by hand, historical sources or evidences of witnesses (or almost witnesses) irrelevant to the theme of analysis, literary and cultural monuments, private letters, and analytical manuscripts. A professional researcher withdraws data from all aspects of human activity in all manifestations.

However, there are special types (political, economical, and military) of information: signed international treaties and accepted governmental laws and regulations. If international treaties and foreign policy documents objectively highlight foreign policy interests, ordinance and regulations correspond to domestic interests and the goals of participators of political and economical processes inside the country (in the opposite case, it is impossible to rest on anything). Thus, it is this information, as well as the records of observing devices, that is fundamental for *understanding* of pragmatic processes.

In the absolute majority of cases, a pragmatic process is empirically irreproducible and, hence, denies an experimental repetition, that is, multiplication, and, therefore, an empirical verification—another principle feature of pragmatic information.

It is self-evident that natural scientific experiments, investigations, and hypotheses can be inaccurate and even contradictory. At the same time, multiplication enables us to verify them. Pragmatic data are accumulated over time. Only a reliably described and correctly analyzed historical experience (in a wide sense) can underlie search for pragmatics laws. In connection with this, historians, sociologists, and economists who arbitrary "dissect" information, can be called the counterfeiters of real pragmatics.

6. The information theory

From the viewpoint of etymology, the word "information" (Latin *informatio*) designating to a massage or explanation implies the interaction (or dialog) between an information source and its consumer. Interaction is the base of human activity, and informational interaction is one of the forms of activity. Hence, data domains and actions must be investigated in parallel with the trends of events, interests giving their birth, words and deeds, and causes and effects. System analysis enables us to obtain important and unexpected results via pure mind. As was said by Bloch [10], p. 23, reality can be best explained according to its causes. In addition, analysis of contradictions can directly indicate sources where missing information or probative base must be sought and "bring historical witnesses to tell even against their will," wrote Bloch [10], p. 23, and, in connection with this, added, "I know questions that should be addressed" to history.

A man, including a desperate individualist, spends his life interacting with the world and people (even Diogenes of Sinope interacted with the Sun, its barrel, and nearest idlers, asking them not to disturb him). From the standpoint of philosophy, human existence involves dialogs with oneself, "the other," and "the others" (i.e., a community). According to the philosophic doctrine of Bakhtin [11], which is shared by Lektorskii [3], pp. 17, 36, 46, the essence and the existence of an individual are inseparably linked with answers on "the appeal of another man," and "another" is the necessary part of the individual ([11], pp. 35–50). Perception and subsequent knowledge arise from interaction with the nature and people, which affect the thoughts and actions of a man.

In the information theory, an informational interaction plays a significant role and is interpreted as the interaction between persons and objects, leading to a change in the database (accumulated information) of one of them ([2], p. 5).

The information transfer technologies have been discussed in Kuznetsov [2], pp. 5, 6. Informational interactions can be divided into three classes (types), namely interactions occurring in artificial (technical) systems (class 1), combined systems (class 2), and natural (living) systems (class 3).

The first class is informational interactions in technical systems: from simplest regulators to global computer networks. The second class contains "living organism-artificial organ," "man-machine," "researcher-inorganic object of investigations," and other interactions. The third class corresponds to informational interactions occurring in the range between molecular genetic levels to social communities. It should be emphasized that the aforementioned types of interactions are tightly coupled during decision-making in the real pragmatics.

In recent years, the unprecedented systems of acquisition, storage, transmission, and analysis of data—computer systems—have been created ([5], p. 91, references). As a result of striking progress in computer technologies, computer systems have become the intellectual communicators, brokers, and competent partners of people in solving the problems of semantics (digital data conversion into conscious information) and pragmatics (data conversion into the knowledge of purposeful activity).

7. Cognitive approach according the evolutionary theory of knowledge

An important feature of informational interactions is linked with the biological aspects of formation of pragmatic knowledge, that is, with the human properties understood as both the tools of world perception (and information obtainment) and the constituents participating in evolution and formation processes. In the latter case, both the biological species and the intellectual and social activities of a man are formed. These problems are thoroughly evaluated in the studies devoted to the evolutionary theory of knowledge (e.g., see [5]).

Biological aspects indicate that external world signals (i.e., objective and subjective data) are perceived by different organs and biological systems (constituents) of a human organism and, thereafter, undergo specific processing, filtering, and changes ([5], pp. 77, 79, 84). In connection with an evolutionary approach, Vollmer indisputably summarizes as follows:

"{Our cognition apparatus is the result of evolution. Subjective cognitive structures correspond to the world due to their formation during adaptation to this real world. They agree (partially) with the real structures because such an agreement enables survival}" ([4], p. 131).

The evolutionary theory of knowledge focuses on that the biological apparatus of a man and its organization were created phylogenetically when people evolved as the biological species. There is no doubt that they are given to each man a priori. The existence of inborn instincts can also be regarded as proven. An ancient problem is whether any man has "inborn concepts" or "inborn forms of cognition." In the metaphorical sense, the issue is whether a man a priori has an intellectual piano or an intellectual composition text book. This problem will be of interest from the view point of determining purposes in the pragmatic analysis technique. The aforesaid is also associated with the correlation between "information" and "knowledge."

Information of different kind, which contains the descriptions of objects, events, and processes ([2], p. 2), is built into the foundation of knowledge and future theory (science). In Section 2, information and informational interactions were discussed as already existing events. Below, the perception and replication (obtainment) of data are considered only if it is necessary to understand the reliability of knowledge and theory.

As was postulated by Gibson [12], perception is an active process of gathering of object (organism) data. This position agrees closely with the information theory. Information carries—technical tools and people—are principally different. Technical tools are known rather well due to their artificial origin. Information can be transferred from an arbitrary technical carrier to computers, that is, represented as computer data. Hence, computer information systems can be assumed to be universal informational equivalents just as gold or money is an equivalent of cost or a medium of exchange.

8. Digital implementation to cognition

When represented with the help of computers, information is the digital implementation of ideas determining an algorithmic (combinatorial) approach. Owing to binary alphabet {0, 1}, words, subsequent algebraic operations, and recursive functions (or algorithms) are formed as though a philosophic ascent from simple to intricate things was carried out, making it possible to computerize all languages, texts, and visual and sound patterns and series.

A discrete set of bits or metasemantic information—computerized data without any sense—can acquire certain values and becomes intelligent and intentional information. This refutes the standpoint according to which representation objects can be formed and exist as a holistic perception.

Partial information or sensation can be considered the separate signs (properties) of observed objects, the certain set of which can characterize (attribute) an object. In practice, this set is used to perform expert examinations. The same principle underlies the uniqueness theorems in mathematics. In this case, a mathematical object satisfying certain conditions (having certain properties) is proved to exists and be unique.

The situation is more complicated if the biological aspects of human perception are investigated. The biological aspects of information obtainment are analyzed exhaustively in Refs. [4, 6, 7, 13, 14] and discussed in Refs. [5, 15]. The illusions of human perception (a Müller Lyer illusion, a Necker cube, a depth illusion, etc.), nonsensory factors, distortions, and instabilities are known, and their research is now being actively per formed. In addition, observation and measurement techniques, which are technical and biological in nature, are inaccurate in principal. In a high magnification microscope, a line segment drawn along the straightest edge of a ruler turns out to be a wavy line. A stretched paint thread, which is used to mark a straight line on a surface (after chalking and stretching, the thread is released, hit the surface, and remains a line of sawcut) is surely not a line segment, but does not differ from the segment by eye. The microscopic image of any straight line is a discrete series of dots instead of a continuous line, a smooth curve displayed by a computer is actually a broken line, etc.

In describing the nonidentity of the environmental reality and the world pattern constructed by each man on its base, R. Bandler and J. Grinder indicate that perception filters can be neurophysiological, social, and individual [16]. These problems are also discussed in Kuznetsov et al. [17].

In addition, the improved information obtainment techniques can cardinally vary our conceptions of the world. Observations with the help of modern high precision instruments indicate that visually immovable and unchangeable objects can vibrate and change their shapes and chemical compositions. In particular, a bright example is a fixed DVD perceived as an immovable flat disk. During observations carried out via laser equipment, this disk exhibits a vibrating curved surface and its shape varies in time.

9. Mathematical theory of errors

Inaccuracies and errors are the properties of any technical device. They are investigated, for example, in the mathematical theory of errors. There are no reasons to attribute the accuracy to biological aspects of perceptions, including a man. What is the meaning of the statement "sensations cannot deceive themselves" and how is interpreted a hazy "argument" of Russel, "In reality, there are no illusions of senses, but data are erroneously interpreted as the signs of things other than themselves" ([3], p. 116)? In the light of the valid physical property of relativism, can "things themselves" be the dependences between the fundamental properties of a substance and the reference (observation) frame? Thus, except for dogmatic reasons, there are no grounds to assert that "an absolute obviousness is a distinctive feature of sensations." Perception can be illusory not only because the activity of mind is conceivable ([3], pp. 115, 116).

10. Theories of Gestalt psychology

A controversial question is whether a human perception is composed of sensations and in what manner ([3], p. 115). The credo of gestalt psychology—a whole is not the sum between constituents, that is, a negative reaction on a psychological structuralism—is beyond any doubt. Among other things, this principle is use to construct all mathematical theories: objects exist not only as things in themselves but also in relations and interactions with each other. However, a proposition that perceptions are always holistic nonatomized images is questionable. Our observing tools and knowledge of a human organism are still very imperfect for making categorical inferences similar to that of gestalt psychologists. However, strictly speaking, an argument is inconsistent when sensations do not exist as the individual images and fragments of perception (elements of perception), at least in this quality, because they are not recognized. Thus, genes, genetic information carriers, are not perceived and cannot be conscious in sensations.

Arguments of Riley [3], p. 116, which were extracted from the ideas of late Wittgenstein, are even more surprising. A man visually perceives concrete things with certain qualities instead of qualities themselves, for example, only objects of the corresponding color rather than the color as a light spectrum—electromagnetic waves of definite waves and frequencies. Hence, sensations are declared as "imaginary objects" with the acquired features of perception and a "categorical error." In connection with this, natural numbers (and, therefore, mathematics based on natural numbers) would be announced as imaginary objects and the categorical error. In contrast to Riley, mathematicians are thought that the separation of numbers and objects is not an error but the discovery made thousands of years ago.

In the context of an evolutionary approach, a significant idea is that evolutionary changes caused by a natural selection lead to the appearance of adaptable sensory systems. As a consequence, all species adequately respond to the environmental features affecting their survival.

Vollmer [4], p. 152, associates information acquisition (or the representation of real objects) with designing in which tree components are taken into account: an object, a projection, and a screen. The designing mechanism has been discussed in

Kuznetsov et al. [5], p. 86. In the Vollmer's scheme, both a "cognitive metaphor" and the term "designing" are successfully employed. However, it goes without saying that metaphors and new terms cannot solve problems, except for those inherent to the representations of adaptors of "language games."

Subjective relativity is capable of distorting the real pragmatics in the description of textual evidences to a greater extent. Hence, the previously noted proposition of Lorenz from *Reversed Side of the Mirror*, which is devoted to the equivalence and interdependence of human physiological systems as the tool of external world perception and the conscious real world ([7], p. 260), is especially actual. Thus, critical analysis of information (or historical sources) is the first and obligatory stage in the construction of the subject theory.

The errors of perception and cognition can also arise from erroneous learning. Let us consider the fragment in the book of M. Goldstein and N. Goldstein, which describes learning of blind persons whose eyesight was recovered in the mature age. To reveal the shapes of geometric figures, the palpation problem is posed instead of the geometrical problem; that is, a tomato is proposed to determine exclusively by color, combining incorrect cooking experiments and "palpation geometry" with the utilitarianism into an inconceivable mismatch of incorrect attainments. If the similar technique is employed to learn experts, we will eat falsifications instead of qualitative products. However, such a situation is definitely encouraging: in our country, learning is not very bad because there are worse processes.

The perception of the world through experience and its cognition were inherent to people long before the formation of knowledge. Information was generated by combining conscious individual data and an informational interaction. A human biological system was formed during an evolutionary process, which required to obtain and estimate (or structurize to some extent) data and, most importantly, comprehend them and apply according to circumstances "here and now" (often instantly) in interactions with the external world. The problems concerning the man's survival as a biological species inevitably led to improvements in information base and behavioral stereotypes (and their subsequent (regular or random) fixation in mind). This phylogenetic aspect of human evolution is most important in the evolutionary theory of knowledge.

In the cognition and interaction processes, a man employs different significant tools: musical, plastic (gestures, dance, and ballet), and visual (painting, graphics, ideograms, and optical images) resources. From the viewpoint of a mathematician, graphics can say no less than words and symbols. Moreover, Zen and Koan practices and language—the most powerful tool whose primary importance was noted by all the cited authors describing the evolutionary theory of knowledge—have not to be forgotten. The linguistic world, where human thought move, in conjunction with the external world provide the foundation of cognition. The correctly used language makes it possible to develop perfected deductive theories, the constituents of scientific cognition. However, the difficulties caused by the development of scientific theories (i.e., the construction of basic concepts, critical analysis of data and semantic knowledge, the validity of inferences, and their interpretation) are beyond the scopes of language problems. These features are known to each mathematician who comprehends the most arduous counterexamples or proofs of problems remained unsolved for centuries or theoreticians in the physical sciences who deal with cosmological models, the problems of quantum mechanics (or field theory), and foundations of theoretical physics as a whole (or any other specialists who solve the complicated technical problems). By a lucky chance, humanitarian dreamers do not suspect these difficulties and assume that the main world problems are the language problems—*sancta simplicitas*.

11. New modern cognitive theories

It is axiomatic that a man does more than creates and improves language and linguistic forms. During the development of new cognitive theories, the linguistics laws (as directives of thought motion) elevate the human mind, and such a process is not connected with any mysticism. However, the man-language, man-object, and language-object interactions do not deserve the new "language idol" instead of idols that were thrown down. (Language and images are synthesized as combination of zeros and unities in computers; that is, is it required to venerate zeros and unities?) Linguists relying on the statement "a man has been created by language" must explain how primitive societies and first public institutions were created by *Homo sapiens* when language did not exist or was more primitive than a man and was less important than gestures (it is necessary not to forget the influence of instruments of labor). Note that children better recognizes patterns than speech.

The process under consideration corresponds to a cognitive process in the three stage scheme proposed by Vollmer (perception-subscientific cognition-scientific cognition). From the viewpoint of the information theory, we deal with transition from nonconscious information of experimental perception to conscious data understood in the context of semantic information, followed by going to semantic knowledge. This process is the first and natural (as historically corresponding to a cognitive process) stage of acquired knowledge (note that the part of modern information is pseudosemantic). The semantic knowledge is the fixed structurized semantic information (from Greek σημαντικοζ signifying having a value).

The semantic knowledge precedes the scientific one. In this case, it is not assumed that the knowledge was concealed in the powerful spirit of Fichte "before all centuries" and patiently waited its birth or was hidden in the world spirit and waited the birth of Hegel to manifests itself. During a purposeful human activity in all possible interactions and biological and social evolutions, the necessity of solving arising problems created both the modern civilization and modern scientific knowledge. The semantic knowledge about the physical world, secrets of handcrafts, human society, and people is more ancient than the scientific knowledge. In the Middle Ages, many discoveries of natural sciences, secrets of handcrafts, and remarkable culinary recipes have been obtained randomly without purposeful investigations. The semantic knowledge involves facts, data, statements, concepts, prejudice, stereotypes, rites, delusions, dogmas, etc.

The prescientific and extrascientific information is called ordinary data and characterized as cognitive, but uncritical. Different types of ordinary knowledge were directives of handcrafts and human behavior and could involve both true and false data. Disordered pro to information can hardly be called the knowledge if its belittling is not the purpose. This is the so called gold carrying ore intended to extract gold. If the human activity is analyzed objectively, the part of knowledge is routinely used in the everyday life and production activity at the level of ordinary instincts and without mental efforts. Hence, the slogan of Maturana and Varela [6], p. 16, 17, "Any action is cognition; any cognition is action," is semicorrected. The action is not always cognition.

According to all cited authors of the publications on the evolutionary theory of knowledge, the human knowledge is greater that the scientific. As was noted by Lektorskii, the scientific knowledge not only contains the prescientific and extrascientific variants but also interacts with them ([3], p. 113). We share this view point and must add that the absolute majority of people has no common with sciences and this undisputable fact cannot be denied by the postulates of Kunh and Feyerabend.

Accurate definition of scientific knowledge is not obligatory. According to M. Castells, the knowledge is "the basic laws of the object domain by which a man can solve arising industrial, scientific, and other problems, that is, facts, concepts, mutual relations, estimates, rules, heuristics (or actual knowledge), and strategies of solutions in this field (or strategic knowledge)" [18]. The knowledge can be divided into declarative (to know what) and procedural (to know how). Declarative knowledge is theoretical because makes it possible to explain the reason of action. Procedural knowledge is pragmatic and corresponds to certain habits. Procedural knowledge can be divided into constructive (to know recipes and instructions) and situational (to act in arising situations). It is possible to separate the third type of knowledge characterizing the culture of the given social system. The behavior of knowledge can implicitly, that is, unallowable for "profane."

The structurization of semantic knowledge, as well as its organization in the human brain (in particular, the known logical level scheme of P. Dilts and G. Bateson: *environment* (when, where, with whom) → *behavior* (what) → *capacities and strategies* (how) → *beliefs and values* (why) → *identity* (who) → *mission* (who and what else)), is discussed in Kuznetsov et al. [17].

Information society is a popular word combination. This term is commonly used in discussions devoted to society, economics, or education.

It is extremely useful to study what meaning has this term when scientists try to describe an information society. In the literature concerned with information society, the number of authors who operate with the undeveloped definitions of the subject is very large. As was emphasized by Webster at the beginning of his study *Information Society Theory* ([19], p. 13), they continuously discuss the features of an information society, but their operational criteria remain uncleared.

The quantitative estimates of the high level of ICT influence on politics and economics are the most popular argument for classifying the modern society as an information community. Competent quantitative analysis performed by F. Muchlup and M. Porat are considered the strong argument in favor of the Porat's inference: the United States has become "the information society the main activity of which is the creation of informational products and services" ([20], p. 32). Analogous statement was postulated by D. Bell in 1973: "we enter into the information society (the synonym of postindustrial society, as was thought D. Bell) when the majority of people are engaged in the information sphere" ([19], p. 21). Well known analytics R. Reich, P. Draker, and M. Castells also assume that the moving force of modern economics is people and their key feature is the use of information ([19], p. 22). Castells begins section *Technology, Society, and Historical Changes* by the words "revolution in information technology covers the entire region of human activity" (however, he explains, "the technology does not predetermine the evolution of society)" ([18], p. 28) and finishes this section as follows: "The modern technological revolution...has appeared and developed during the global restructurization of capitalism and is an important tool of restructurization. Thus, a new society born due to this transformation is both capitalistic and informational."

Webster note that "the majority of definitions of an information society are based on quantitative characteristics" and separates five definitions associated with the identification of innovations: technological, economical, coupled with the sphere of employment, spatial, and cultural. Emphasizing that the grounds of these definitions are the statement that quantitative changes in the information sphere have led to the formation of a qualitatively new social structure—information society, and the reasoning that our society is informational due to an increase in the volume of information and the appearance of information society is caused by the appearance of new information technologies ([19], p. 17), he criticizes this questionable structure.

12. Quantitative approaches to knowledge

Indicating the debatableness of the quantitative approach, Webster writes in the first chapters ([19], p. 19): "{The main problem is that hidden subjective interpretations, as well as estimation statements related to the construction of categories and the incorporations and eliminations of an informational sector, stand behind the statistical tables, which must confirm the objectivity of proofs.}"

As a consequence, the principal problems are the unreliable foundation and structure of all quantitative approaches. Without analyzing the arguments of the different authors, we can indicate that the implementations of informfile ideas and the release out of the industrial society have led to the replacement of the Great Britain (the nineteenth century) and USA (the twentieth century) workshops of the world with the China workshop of the world (the twenty-first century).

Webster thoroughly discusses and denies the Bell's concept, engages in polemics with Castells, but must admit that information is the fundamental factor in the modern economics ([19], p. 72). Let us consider its role in the ICTs of the existing world and in the theoretical knowledge (which is of equal importance).

Although many intellectuals and politics interpret new technologies as the newest idols with keys to progress and healing, the situation is more complicated.

During historical evolution, none of the technologies was considered the determining factor of our society. The discovery of a wheel, the domestication of a horse, and the inventions of a metallurgical process, a steam engine, or a lifting vehicle (very important inventions) do not imply that "horse" or "steam" society has arisen.

Owing to the ICT influence on different aspects of current life, numerous investigations of an influence process are performed. Below, we do not consider the current political problems: globalization, a growth in ICT influence (and, therefore, national sovereignty restrictions), class problems of a traditional political economy (the works of Shiller), information distortions and its manipulations for political purposes (the favorite topic of Yu. Khabermas), but focuses on philosophic problems.

Coinciding with the substantiated inferences of Webster (i.e., the appearance and development of unprecedented ICTs, the sharply increased amount of information, the growth of its influence on the current activity, society organization, etc. cannot be regarded as the features of the new type of the society of the new epoch ([19], p. 80)), we must indicate the occurred principle changes.

It is accepted that a distinctive feature of the existing "information society" is the information transformation into the good. "Knowledge is created to be sold and consumed to acquire cost in the new product," declares Lyotard [21], p. 19 (it is clear that he does not know the Pushkin's expression: "Inspiration is not sold, but a manuscript can be sold"). G. Shiller has assumed that the information revolution is hallmarked with the continuously sharpened inequality (the point at issue). However, the information and knowledge transformation into the valuable product is scarcely the new process. The secrets of silk production, violin manufacturers, bell molding and other corporate secrets (including culinary), which were state secrets, military technologies, etc. always estimated higher than gold. Mongolian vanquishers and Tamerlane took care of captive artisans. In the Middle Ages, books were very expensive even after the discovery of paper. Beginning at least from the thirteenth century, both technological and legal literacies were valued highly. After Guttenberg discovered book printing, the number books printed in Europe for 50 years substantially exceeded the number books written for several preceding centuries; that is, the revolution has occurred. Hence, this society could be called informational (in addition, this was the period of great geographical discoveries). Thus, from the viewpoint of aspects discussed above, it is necessary to note the continuity of our epoch instead of its exceptionality.

As to postmodernistic (proofless) prophecies that the entire data and science will be transformed into a commercial shop, they will fail. Mercenariness is an important, but not sole, aspect or motif. Even ancient Roman understood that *spiritus ubi vult spirum* (the spirit moves in an arbitrary direction). Scientific and technological investigations always required financing. However, many investigations and discoveries have been carried out without proper payments and even contrary to mercantile interests. Moreover, profitable discoveries were not often supposed to be gainful.

However, the high data transmission rates, which have led to the new types of business; the information dissemination freedom, which has strongly hampered its concealment; and the state authority functioning with the help of Internet technologies were not observed previously. The Castells' attention to informational networks ([18], Ch. 3–5) and their constructive and destructive functions in the society is undoubtedly justified.

Intellectual aspects are as important as political economical relations. According to F. Webster, "although the theoretical knowledge priority is little discussed in the information society theories, there are many grounds to interpret this property as a distinctive feature of modernity." In addition, it is proposed without proofs that "it is possible to prove that the theoretical knowledge plays a key role in the modern society in contrast to the preceding epoch with dominant practical and situational knowledge" ([19], p. 38). "This knowledge is formalized in texts and transferred mainly by learning" ([19], p. 39). In addition, Webster kindly cites D. Bell who assures us that industrial revolutions were performed by "talented dreamer indifferent to sciences and the fundamental laws underlying discoveries." It is likely that Bell both observed the flashes of inspirations of dreamers and penetrated into their thoughts. The current situation differs in that "innovations are initiated by principle knowledge; their initiation clearly manifests itself in the field of science and technology (note that these principles can be understood by a small number of experts)" ([19], p. 38). Let imagine yourselves that Aristotle's, Euclid's, Galilei's, and Newton's crowds roamed the streets in the previous years. It is of interest whether anyone can guarantee that the current dreamers will not call liars in 200 years.

Note that F. Webster uncritically expounds the views of D. Bernar and N. Shter [19], p. 163.

We agree with Webster's concept about the high significance of theoretical knowledge and the remark "in our time...the theoretical knowledge underlies many political decisions and debates" ([19], p. 39), but the words "in our time" are obscure. It seems that *State* of Plato, *Politicians* of Aristotle, *De Cavitate Dei* of St. Augustine, *De Monarchia* of Dante, *Prince* of Macki Avelli, *Mahaprajnaparamita sutra* of Nagarjuna, and *Conversations and Statements* of K'ung Fu tzu (Confucius) and other publications prepared his successors were not written or they weakly affected the minds of politicians. It is clear that there is no need to remember the influence of political and economical doctrines, which "became the material force and seized the masses."

We also assume that accents must be changed. "Theoretical knowledge has become the defining feature of our world," was written by Webster [19], p. 40.

The problem must be posed in the following manner: *what* (in the qualitative sense) theoretical knowledge has become the defining feature of our world.

13. Post-modern approaches to cognitive psychology

The orthodox Marxism-Leninism crisis and the USSR decomposition had unexpected consequences. At the beginning of postmodernism, which is called both an intellectual process and our everyday life ([19], p. 312), postmodernists interested in culture and art. However, in the last two decades of the twentieth century, they have passed to total generalizations (it is rather surprising because they refused all total theories). As was interpreted by postmodernists, the collapse of the so-called socialist system confirms that not only "great statements" (a bright metaphor of Lyotard)—proofless doctrines pretended to the generality and infallibility—but also other theories aspired to the authenticity and truth are inconsistent. They began with correctly criticizing the precarious concepts of aforementioned theories, such as "progress," "humanism," and "civilization development." (In general, starting with Hegel, many philosophers better criticize and deny than create.) Thereafter, it was indicated that the dogmas of Enlightenment philosophers (i.e., the laws exist in the historical process and the political being and actions of people is rational and understandable as the a priori truth) cannot be accepted. However, postmodernists simultaneously threw the child out with bathwater. Let us briefly analyze this situation because the postmodernism intended to play the role of the main social philosophic direction of modern times.

Postmodernistic arguments rely on four principal statements. Firstly, it is assumed that the adequate and objective description and analysis of the historical process and humanitarian world are impossible. A man and political existence are declared to be incognizable (because the course of history discredits such attempts).

The second principal statement is more radical: there no reality and truth due to the "multiplicity of representations," but imaginary meanings are possible.

The third statement is pseudopositive: the place of the reality is occupied by empty information (various symbols and linguistic games).

Fourthly, in the opinion of postmodernists, the unavoidable subjectivity of a researcher is caused by both personal subjective and political commitments. Its propagandistic purpose is the event orientation in the definite direction by means of arbitrary extrapolations.

Let us consider these problems. Let us begin with the second (deepest) statement. Indeed, the truth multiplicity is an important problem. The truth multiplicity proved by mathematicians in the twentieth century (e.g., Indian philosopher assumed that the truth multiplicity is a self-evident fact and denied the objective and absolute truths ([22], p. 39)) resembles the postulation of a single absolute truth in the West philosophy and is the principal discovery. The simplest example is alternative geometries. It is firmly ascertained that the axiom of parallels, as well as its negation, is compatible with the axiomatics of absolute geometry. Similar to alternative geometries, the standard axiomatics of the theory of Zermelo-Fraenkel (ZF) sets is compatible with both the axiom of choice (AC) and its negation. In other words, ZF sets can be extended both to theory (ZF + AC) and to theory (ZF +? AC). However, each theory will have its own drawbacks ([11], p. 177). In addition, the well-known continuum hypothesis (to solve the continuum problem, investigations have been performed for almost a century) turns out to be independent of ZF sets. The possibility of existing of Lebesgue non-measurable sets (not having the length or area), as well as the possibility of non-existing, is considered in Jech [23], Ch. 20. *Here, the problem is solved in the completely opposite manner*: several truths are possible (however, only in the perfect theories with infinite basic positions).

In this case, there are no contradictions. In any theory, the contradiction is admissible. The truth multiplicity and inconsistency are completely different things. The problem can be solved by two methods. The first of them is to investigate the sources and grounds of alternative theories, as is done in mathematical logic, for example, in the proof theory. The other method is to rely on contradictions. In this case, postmodernists are not pioneers: "contradiction is the source of any motion and vitality; something moves, has motivations, and is active only due to an internal contradiction," Hegel [24], Book 2, p. 65. The problem is hampered by continuous mixing of contradictions and contrapositions, which was predicted by Kant [25] (this work was underestimated by his successors). The contradiction was previously related to the magic word “dialectics.” At present, the magic word is “relativism.”

Analyzing postmodernistic arguments of adequacy and truth in the context of the correlated first and second statements (in Ch. 9), Webster highlights their initial propositions:

Each representation and description of the reality is mainly falsified (“truth versions”). This proposition is called by the godlessly disturbed term “relativism,” which was borrowed from theoretical physics. Hence, search for authenticity is senseless.

The reality is replaced with symbols, linguistic games, and unreal and empty estimates. Events occur in the world where “the concept of reality” is eliminated (the scheme of J. Baudrillard).

Accepting contradictions inherent to the society as a whole and each person, we must forget about the existence of true I.

In addition, it is necessary to consider postmodernistic concepts of the practice of these linguistic games (see Lyotar*d, @Scientific Knowledge Pragmatics*, Ch. 7), which is interpreted as a learning process (i.e., the teacher-student process). Since the directives of learning have a certain degree of acceptability, they are regarded to be “scientific.” “The truth” and “the scientific content” of directives are determined by the resolutions of the narrow specialized isolated community of experts. Lyotard calls this community “the scientific institute” (such communities were referred to as sects in the days of old). “The truth of a directive and the competence of an expert depend mainly on the approval of group of expert with equal competences” ([21], pp. 62–63).

In this case, all phenomena become reversed. The truth of phenomena is determined by checked observations and measurements, rather than resolutions and approvals of a certain community. The observations and measurements are primary, and the resolutions are their consequences. The geocentric system will not be true due to the resolutions of the scientific institute even after “the name of Trismegist Aristotle.” At the same time, this system is true not only because of the approval by the Copernicus scientific institute, which “announced that planets have circular trajectories. The institute assumes that it can prove its announcements. On the other hand, any statement related to the same expert is eliminated if it is inverse or contradictory” ([21], p. 62). However, the reasons of elimination are unintelligible. As was declared by Webster, “the TRUTH” is replaced with “the truth multiplicity” and there is no commonly used method of selection among the components of this set. As was affirmed by Lyotard ([26], p. 66) the truth is the issue of selection (i.e., only the accepted residue remains). To give a complete picture, it should be said: according to the order of Lyotard in 1988.

To corroborate and justify the elimination of the reality, surprising assertions about freedom are used (by the way, how to philosophize without the freedom). “After making a decision on the essence of truth, we easily come to tyranny” ([19], p. 319). Then, the principal total tyranny is mathematics, and mathematicians are slaves. In this case, without lapsing into tyranny and determining the criteria of estimation and selection, it is impossible to find whether Mahatma Gandhi is better than Hitler. However, postmodernists, one and all, do not want to live under the control of Hitler or Stalin.

As postmodernists deny the truth, it would be correct to say that “the multiplicity of senses” (or, simply, “the multiplicity of subjective, erroneous, and contradictory senses”) instead of “the multiplicity of truths.” The reason is the uniqueness of researchers of the humanitarian world and history. What if natural sciences could be created by automatic machines or clowns? “Postmodernism denies all claims to the reality: nothing can be true and authentic because everything is falsified” ([21], p. 325). Why postmodernists announce that researchers of the humanitarian world are falsifiers? Why they (in contrast to specialists of natural sciences) tend toward falsification?

Why they demonstrate contempt both to other scientists and, strictly speaking, to themselves? These questions have no clear answers. It is likely that other purposes and means exist and, in addition, other requirements and criteria are imposed.

There are the other, absolutely correct, reasons: the subjectivity of observation tools (in the first place, a man as a biological tool of observations) and the subjectivity of evidences. They have already been discussed in the context of pragmatic information.

However, it is necessary to make an absolutely different inference: any pragmatic investigation must be preceded by thorough critical analysis accompanied by the detection of possible contradictions and their elimination or the explanation the impossibility of elimination. However, all occurs contrariwise: facts are arbitrary analyzed or remained unverified and proofs, including arguments, are replaced with declarations. In natural sciences, such a practice is inapplicable.

Why the humanitarian world is senseless and unreal? Why the actions of its objects are unreason able, contradictory, and incognizable, as is announced by postmodernists in their total extrapolations from culture to the whole pragmatism? The fauna is real and is the subject of science. The behavior of unreasonable animals is characterized by the directivity and consistency. Biology has revealed the behavioral laws of animals. Why a man is defective even in comparison with animals?

Although sociologists and historians are in extremely intricate situation, biologists and their evolution undergo greater difficulties. It can be thought that the quantum physics, cosmology, and genetics problems are simpler. The negation of the reality and truth is an ordinary dogma, which is not substantiated but is the indulgence of the lack of knowledge and skill. However, if "there is no reality, but the language," and the unreal world around us is created by information, what is the subject of postmodernistic investigations? Is it possible that they investigate themselves?

Let us only imagine that houses and bridges, air crafts, and nuclear reactors are created on the basis of postmodernistic principles. Generally speaking, if postmodernists are collected on the separate territory and live according to their principles, the natural selection will rapidly lead to their extinction (God forbid, we do not wish it).

It is undoubted that constructive analysis is much better than postmodernistic intellectual groans and round dances of general phrases and abstruse terms. However, for this purpose, the pragmatic analysis laws must be determined and pragmatic theories must be developed.

The reliability and completeness of information are very important factors. Postmodernists correctly indicate modern "informational hazards." As was noted by Lyotard, information is not only gathered and analyzed but also concealed and distorted due to propagandistic reasons. Indeed, we drown in the sea of symbols, ceasing to designate anything. Rozak [19], pp. 34–36, asks whether the increasing volume of information leads to the higher informativity of citizens. Thus, there appear two problems: data obtainment and their rejection. Therefore, information must be complete and properly structurized.

In this case, we encounter some problems and cardinally new possibilities, which make it possible to say about "the information society." All archives are being successfully digitized. It seems probable that this process will be finished in the nearest future. Thereafter, all the materials of natural and humanitarian sciences will be generally available in the Internet. In this case, an end will be put to the absolutely vicious practice of rational minds to select somewhat important parts from data according to their hierarchy of values, arbitrary concealing or distorting other parts. Then, any researcher and "scientific institute" (according to Lyotard) will be able to validate the completeness and consistency of the database used to construct one or another concept, thereby checking the perfection of foundations.

Thus, each of us can validate the perfection of substantiations. In this case, the conception inferences must be confirmed by strict (error free and complete) *proofs*, which must be correspond to definite true theorem instead of general statements comprising round dances of general phrases sanctified by a popular expert, *ism*th, or a political order. In addition, it can be checked that the concept has no contradictions with the known facts. As a consequence, intellectual dreamers will not mislead an ordinary leader and themselves.

The correctly structurized scientific part of the Internet (together with public libraries) will be "the keeper of facts" the significance of which was highlighted by Webster, Phillips, and Moser [19], p. 254. Thus, it will be possible (by means of the power of thought) to enter into the epoch of the substantiated "theoretical knowledge" of new technologies and real pragmatics.

Knowledge applicable to the real pragmatics—purposeful human activity—is of special significance. From the pragmatic standpoint, there are good natural reasons to assume that knowledge is information capable of generating an action stimulating comprehension [27].

In practice, knowledge can be considered intellectual assets, which can provide and provides real dividends to companies: patents, copyrights, the knowledge and professional quantities of specialists, trademarks, a client base, the network of loyal providers and partners, the culture of innovation implementation, a corporative memory and databases, the quality of working procedures, etc. According to utilitarianism, this is an important factor and the challenging motif of an efficient and successful economical activity.

14. Principles of professional knowledge

The professional knowledge involves the following aspects:

Cognitive knowledge ("to know that"): the mastering of a basic discipline. Specialists attain a high level of skill due to intensive learning and certification.

Applied skill ("to know how"): "book learning" is transformed into efficient execution. The ability of employing the rules belonging to a definite discipline to solve existing complicated problems. This is most widespread professional level leading to the creation of valuable products.

System understanding ("to know why"): the deep understanding of the entire system of mutual relations and causes and effects underlying a definite discipline.

Personal motivation of creative work ("to want to know why") embraces will, motivation, and aiming for success.

Together with creation and maintenance of intellectual capital, it is necessary to abandon certain obsolete and inappropriate types of knowledge. Therefore, the problem concerning knowledge acquisition and management is posed. The knowledge management is the key component of scientific and industrial activities in the mordent society.

The knowledge management has two trends: efficiency, the use of knowledge to increase productivity by increasing the speed and decreasing expenses, and innovations intended to create new products and services, new enterprises, and new business processes.

According to the investigations of Liebowitz and Beckmann ([28], p. 76) the knowledge management can be divided into eight stages.

From the tactical standpoint, a knowledge management process is accepted to divide into four stages: information gathering (acquisition), application, learning, and dissemination. The basic problem is the development of system indices used to estimate the advantages of investments in a knowledge base. Practical recommendations and the structurization and systematization processes of knowledge management are discussed in Bukowitz and Williams [29].

Since the data exchange speed and the technological innovation rate have increased, it is necessary to update the traditional educational system. In the knowledge and human resource management and professional technical education and training, the dominant position is occupied by the competence approach, which integrates education and training into practice (e.g., see [30]) and involves both a competence and a functional competency, that is, the capability of demonstrating its competence.

15. Trends to competence approach

The competence approach as a whole comprises three trends. In the *behavioral approach* (an American tradition), the main attention is devoted to a high motivation and an efficient operation during the interaction of a man and an environment. The *functional approach* (a British tradition) is based on the functional competency in which knowledge, comprehension, and skills are employed according to the specified standards, including the problem solution and compliance with varying requirements. The *multidimensional and holistic approach* (France, Germany, and Great Britain) deals with knowledge, skills, and comprehension (action), which are selected as the constituents of the structurally complicated competence model.

Competences are accepted to classify into three directions: cognitive, social, and personal competences. The Council of Europe has defined five groups of major social competences, which "must be attributed to young Europeans," as is reported by Hutmacher in [31].

However, in parallel with utilitarian and practical problems, which can be regarded as technological problems, an equivalent attention must be devoted to the following principal issues: How the reliable scientific knowledge is selected among the pragmatic knowledge; what is the necessary tool in "distinguishing between truth and conspicuity" (Kant), and how knowledge is transformed into scientific theories.

Semantic information structurization is an obligatory initial stage, which precedes the semantic knowledge transformation into a scientific theory. The selection problems concerned with the rapidly increasing flow of new data require the cardinal reconstruction of the Internet, i.e., its division into free and professional parts. The free part is restricted only by legal requirements. The professional part must involve portals, the number of which can be increased according to expert council decisions. The existing situation, in which much time is spent to find desired data (their reliability is unknown) among garbage collections, is inadmissible.

16. Conclusions

At present, the amount of technical instruments is high enough (much greater than in the previous century) to implement adequate observations and measurements of the humanitarian world. In addition, it is interesting to know the correlation between the reality and the postmodernistic world, where "nothing can be true and authentic because everything is falsified." ("It is very interesting that you have no things I requested from you," was said by Voland in the Bulgakov's novel *Master and Margarita*, Ch. 3.)

How important is the question about the world in which politicians, economists, and intellectuals play political linguistic games without our participation. Is it good that the life and philosophy begin and end by linguistic games? Probably, there is a need to change existing guidelines and target designations compelling us to live in the world where proportions between an external form and the content (thought) are violated. Must we adore the newest technologies? Can we become wiser after the obtainment of a new electronic device?

What must determine pragmatic plans, decisions, and human actions? In the biological sense, the efficient behavior is the result of multicentury evolution and millions of tests and errors. In the social, political, and economical senses, a humanitarian community cannot allow such expanses. How pragmatic theories are created? What underlies their grounds? What is the pragmatic analysis procedure? What inferences can be regarded as reliable? In addition, there is a need to ascertain whether scientific investigations and strategic plans are prophecies or something like "ku ka re ku" in the postmodernistic style.

To what degree the scientifically established laws of the physical world can be assumed to be hypothetical? Is it successful that a cognitive scheme is classified as the "hypothetical realism" (Lorenz, D. Campbell, and G. Vollmer)? Is it possible to assert that "each hypothesis is an intuitive guesswork"? Is it true that D.I. Mendeleev fell asleep and the periodic system of elements was his intuitive guesswork in a dream?

Another important problem is related to the a priori forms of cognition. The existence of congenital instincts seems to be proven. Are there innate concepts and hypothesis? It may be that cognition is a simple remembering of them. However, great Hellenes did not know about basic arithmetical symbols—modern Indian numbers and the radix notation. Moreover, they have no fundamental concepts about motion of celestial bodies. The "congenital concept" of an irrational segment appeared many years ago and led to the revolution in ancient mathematics. At the same time, the "congenital concept" of an irrational number was not created by Newton, Leibniz, and Euler. The fundamental concept of space (more exactly, spaces) was not formulated even by Kant and Hegel. The "congenital concepts" of mathematical logic were born only at the end of the twentieth century. Note that many "con genital physical concepts" have not been created up to the twentieth century. Thus, the problem under consideration remains unexplained.

The aforesaid is important to determine the correct technique if pragmatic analysis, the variant of which has been proposed in Refs. [32, 33] and called conceptual analysis.

Vollmer was emphasized that scientific knowledge is based on observations and experiments. He correctly assumes that its attributes are critical analysis of information, the formulation and checkout of hypothesis, and the use of cognitive models and deductive conclusions. However, an especially significant aspect of pragmatic scientific knowledge is the construction of pragmatic theories. The architectonics of pragmatic theories, analysis of philosophy, and the results of analytical history will be discussed in the subsequent study.

Author details

Oleg Evgenevich Baksansky
Lebedev Physical Institute of the Russian Academy of Sciences, Moscow, Russia

*Address all correspondence to: obucks@mail.ru

References

[1] Aristotel S. Works in 4 Vol. Moscow: Mysl'; 1976. pp. 75-76. [in Russian]

[2] Kuznetsov NA. Information interaction in techno logical living systems. Russian Journal Informatsionnye Protsessy. 2001;**1**:1-9

[3] Lektorskii VA. Epistemology Classical and Not Classical. Moscow: Editorial URSS; 2009 [in Russian]

[4] Vollmer G. Evolutionare Erkenntnistheorie: Angeborene Erkenntnisstrukturen im Kontext von Biologie, Psychologie, Linguistik, Philosophie und Wissenschaftstheorie. Stuttgart: Hirzel; 1981 (Moskow, 1998)

[5] Kuznetsov NA, Baksanskii OE, Grech ishkina NA. Origin of knowledge: Backgrounds and foundations. Russian Journal Informatsionnye Protsessy. 2007;7(1):72-92

[6] Maturana HR, Varela FH. Tree of Knowledge. Biological Roots of Human Understanding. Boston: Shambhala; 1987 (Moscow: Progress Traditsiya; 1999) [in Russian]

[7] Lorenz K. Die Ruckseite des Spiegels: Versuch einer Naturgeschichte menschlichen Erkennens. Munchen: Piper; 1973 (Moscow: Respublika; 1998)

[8] Martin NFG, England JW. Mathematical The ory of Entropy. Reading: Addison Wesley; 1981 (Moscow: Mir; 1988)

[9] Barr Hillel Y, Carnap R. Semantic information. British Journal for the Philosophy of Science. 1953;**4**(4):7

[10] Bloch M. Apologie pour l'histoire ou Metier d'historien. Paris: Armand Colin; 1949 (Moscow: Mir; 1986)

[11] Bakhtin MM. Aesthetics of Verbal Creation. Moscow: Iskusstvo; 1979 [in Russian]

[12] Gibson JJ. The Ecological Approach to Visual Perception. Boston: Houghton Mifflin; 1979 (Moscow: Progress; 1988)

[13] Schiffman HR. Sensation and Perception. An Integrated Approach. New York: Wiley and Sons; 2001 (St. Petersburg: Piter; 2003)

[14] Simon H. The Sciences of the Artificial. Cambridge, MA: MIT Press; 1969 (Moscow: Editorial URSS; 2004)

[15] Kuznetsov NA, Baksanskii OE, Grech ishkina NA. Modeling of intellectual activities: touch input in cognitive system. Russian Journal Informatsionnye Protsessy. 2007;7:432-474

[16] Bandler R, Grinder J. The Structure of Magic: A Book about Language and Therapy. Palo Alto, CA: Science and Behavior Books; 1975 (Moscow: Al'yans; 2001)

[17] Kuznetsov NA, Baksanskii OE, Grech ishkina NA. Fundamental importance of informatics in contemporary scientific picture of world. Russian Journal Informatsionnye Protsessy. 2006;7:81-109

[18] Castells M. The Information Age: Economy, Society and Culture. Oxford: Blackwell; 1996 (Moscow: GU-VShE; 2000)

[19] Webster F. Theories of the Information Society. London: Routledge; 1995 (Moscow: Aspekt Press; 2004)

[20] Porat MU. Communication policy in an information society. In: Robinson GO, editor. Communications for Tomorrow. New York: Praeger; 1978. pp. 3-60

[21] Lyotard JF. The Postmodern Condition, A Report on Knowledge. Manchester: Manchester Univ. Press; 1984 (St. Petersburg: Aleteja; 1998)

[22] Kanaeva NA. Problem of Terminal Knowledge in India. Moscow: Vost. Literatua; 2002

[23] Jech TJ. Lectures in Set Theory, with Particular Emphasis on the Method of Forcing. Berlin: Springer Verlag; 1971 (Moscow: Mir; 1973)

[24] Hegel GWF. Die Wissenschaft der Logik. Nurnberg; 1812-1813 Moscow: MSU; 1970

[25] Kant I. Versuch den Begriff der negativen Gröossen in der Weltweisheit einzufuhren. Köonigsberg: Johann Jacob Kanter; 1763 (AK II, 165-204)

[26] Kant I. Attempt to introduce the concept of negative magnitudes into philosophy. In: Collected Works in 8 Vols. Vol. 2. Moscow: Mysl'; 1993-1996. [in Russian]

[27] Lyotard JF. The Difference: Phases in Dispute. Manchester: Manchester Univ. Press; 1988

[28] Rumizen MC. The Complete Idiot's Guide to Knowl edge Management. Indianapolis, IN: Alpha; 2002 (AST, Moscow, 2004). Available from: www.koism.rags.ru/publ/articles/26.php

[29] Bukowitz W, Williams R. Knowledge Management Fieldbook. Old Tappan, NJ: Prentice Hall; 1999 (Moscow: Infra; 2002)

[30] Raven J, Stephenson J, editors. Competence in the Learning Society. New York: Peter Lang; 2001 (Moscow: Kogito Tsentr; 2002)

[31] Hutmacher W. Key competencies for Europe. In: Report of the Symposium Berne, Switzerland, Mar 27-30, 1996. Strasburg: Council for Cultural Co operation (CDCC)/Secondary Education for Europe; 1997

[32] Zholkov CY. Available from: http://www.gubkin.ru/personal_sites/

[33] Zholkov SY. On laws of society and history I. Alma Mater–Vestnil Vysshei Shkoly. 2010;**2**:16-26

Chapter 3

The Role of Self-Efficacy and Cognitive Behaviour Therapy in Forming Prosocial Behaviour

Rosmawati Mohamad Rasit and Siti Zuhrah Che Ab Razab

Abstract

Prosocial value can be associated with the positive behaviours that are commonly practised in the socio-surrounding of a civilised community, for example, the action of helping, loving and developing empathy with each other. The formation of the prosocial behaviour also has a connection with one's self-efficacy. The individual's mastery of his or her self-efficacy can contribute to the differences in how he or she is behaving. All of the ethical values in every religion explain life as revolving around helping one another and living peacefully in society. The effort of helping based on the concerns towards other people could be the motivational factors that are closely related to the prosocial behaviour. Having positive personality traits and then backed with a sound religious belief ingrain the necessary moral compass that guides a person into behaving in ways that are considered society-friendly. Meanwhile, media roles depending on the content are capable of propagating decent values among the larger mass. Generally speaking, these factors are sufficient in educating and nurturing normal individuals to attain better self-efficacy. However, on an earnest ground considering individuals who suffer from a low level of self-efficacy, which resulted in antisocial behaviour, a more structured and empirical psychological intervention needs to be administered.

Keywords: prosocial, behaviour, self-efficacy, religion, community

1. Introduction

Self-efficacy is a trait where one can make a sound judgement about his or her own decision. An individual who trusts him or herself is considered of having good self-efficacy. Therefore, self-efficacy is a crucial factor in creating a harmonious society through the demonstration of ethical behaviour. Bandura [1] argues that an individual who possesses a high level of self-efficacy can achieve personal success as well as behave positively. On the contrary, a person with a low level of self-efficacy is less successful and less confident in achieving the goals set. According to Eisenberg et al. [2], the existence of the *perceived self-efficacy* as a factor in social learning cognitive is related to the *emphatic* efficacy perception, which is also related to prosocial behaviour. Thus, self-efficacy serves as a critical factor in how far a person can involve him or herself with the feedback from other people.

However, every person has a different personality trait. The diversity of human personality becomes the determiners of prosocial behaviour. Penner et al. [3]

suggest that those who have a prosocial personality have more readiness to help others and are more emphatic. Based on a study by Penner et al. [3], the *Helpfulness* factor serves as the predictor that explains prosocial behaviour better than the *Other-oriented Empathy* factor. Penner et al. [3] argumentation involves *helping*, which has a strong link with self-efficacy than the environmental skills mastery. This link explains that someone who is consistently involved in prosocial behaviour does so because he or she is doing something for him or herself, not only because of his or her contributions to others.

Meanwhile, according to Norenzayan and Shariff [4], a society that practices a more religious life tends to behave more prosocially due to the understanding of the concept of God. The studies on the relationship between prosocial behaviour and religion explain about the religious influence on the prosocial value in a society such as simplifying a behaviour that can benefit others [4], teaching about compassion [5], volunteering to help as well as acting non-aggressively [6] when coming into contact with the daily routine.

According to NICE Guideline on Diagnosis, Assessment and Management of Harmful Drinking and Alcohol Dependence published by the British Psychological Society and the Royal College of Psychiatrists, NICE [7], psychological interventions consist of a broad spectrum that is subjected to the underpinning theoretical models. They are classified under several approaches such as behavioural, cognitive, psychodynamic, humanistic, systemic, motivational, disease, and social and environmental. In relation to nurturing higher level of self-efficacy among individuals who suffer from low-level self-efficacy so that they can behave more prosocially, cognitive behavioural therapy is considered as a two-in-one approach to address the issues based on the assumptions that cognition has a significant influence on humans' emotional and behavioural impediment [8]. This section centres on a brief discussion on psychological intervention, particularly cognitive behavioural therapy, which is one of the intervention approaches that are empirically supported and evidence-based to see convincing results [9].

2. Self-efficacy

Self-efficacy is a concept that can be linked to the extent of control that a person has over the situation in his or her life. A person with a high level of self-efficacy is someone who thinks positively, charismatic, courageous and persistence. Therefore, self-efficacy becomes a factor that leads to the behaviour of a person. Bandura [10] discusses the concept of self-efficacy, which also influences behaviour. Self-efficacy can be explained as a person's trust or judgement on the faculty and competence of his or herself to carry out actions to achieve specific goals set [1, 10–12].

In other words, self-efficacy is the inherent belief of the extent of the ability to act based on the faculty within oneself. Self-efficacy can influence a person's performance achievement [10] whether it is at a peak or otherwise. It means the level of self-efficacy is capable of influencing more excellent contribution to work performance compared to those with a low level of self-efficacy. This self-competence becomes a crucial factor in the cognitive, motivation and health aspect formation process [1]. The individuals who have a high level of self-efficacy exhibit characteristics of those among the successful and consistent in their strategic planning.

Therefore, we can see that individuals with high self-efficacy possess the determination and readiness to sacrifice for the benefit of others. They reason and can accept challenges with high determination. It is the opposite of individuals with low self-efficacy. They will avoid doing strenuous work and always see life challenges

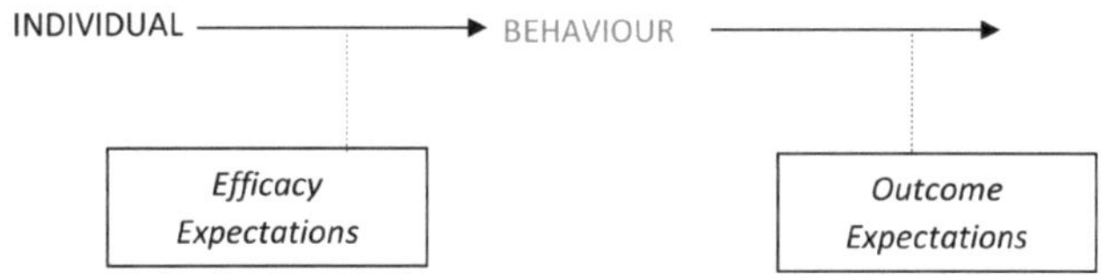

Figure 1.
Diagram of the representation of the differences between efficacy expectations and outcome expectations. Source: Bandura [1].

as problems that haunt their lives. These individuals are incapable of accepting the burden, and in life, they often end up in despair. They are incapable of controlling themselves with negative thoughts and blame others for what has happened in their life. According to Bandura [1], the capability to master good cognitive and thinking skills will enable the control of matters that can affect one's life.

Bandura [1] differentiates between *efficacy expectations* and *outcome expectations* (**Figure 1**). Bandura [1] places self-efficacy as efficacy expectations. *Efficacy expectations* involve the perception towards the ability of the self in determining the expected actions. Meanwhile, *outcome expectations* serve as self-estimation regarding the behaviours performed that will result in specific outcomes. Through *efficacy expectations*, an individual is capable of evaluating an action performed whether it is good, bad, precise or otherwise. *Efficacy expectations* portray the ideal self-evaluation that can be achieved, whereas the *outcome expectations* achievement depends on an individual's endurance in ensuring that the wish is fulfilled [1]. This mean, an individual can have realistic *efficacy expectations*, which is hoped can be materialised; however, the *outcome expectation*s will become unrealistic if the hope is too high from the actual expected results.

Therefore, an individual with high-efficacy expectations is confident in being able to carry out actions that are suitable for the situational demands. Meanwhile, the realistic outcome expectations that are aligned with the faculty of the self will cause the individual to work hard and is capable of achieving the goals set. Self-efficacy becomes the mediator that can determine individuals' behaviour, whereas the individuals play the role of controlling actions through self-control assessment. The self-control mechanism enables a person to set realistic *outcome expectations* that are aligned with their ability and faculty. Self-efficacy is closely linked to excellence in achieving good performance, which is assessed as cognitive determinants. Muhammad Awais [13] argues about self-efficacy that it is capable of providing the measurement regarding one's personality aspect that involves motivation and trust. Meanwhile, according to Eklund et al. [14], individuals who have a high level of self-efficacy have better prosocial value and are more popular.

3. Prosocial behaviour

Helpfulness trait has become the practice of today's society. The need to offer help is not limited to those we know but also strangers. Similarly, the caring attitude towards other people's welfare in a sincere manner that hopes for nothing in return has become a social practice within societal life environment. These traits form a prosocial value that leads to prosocial behaviour. According to Hastings et al. [15], prosocial behaviour is a form of behaviour that is voluntarily performed in the attempt to benefit others. It is a response that is performed proactively and reactively towards other people's needs in the attempt to promote healthier social life. Therefore, volunteering activities should be nurtured as a society's responsibility towards a healthy and prosperous life. It can also encourage social responsibility in shaping prosocial attitude among the local community.

Prosocial behaviour is a positive behaviour that is the opposite of the antisocial behaviour as the negative behaviour. Prosocial behaviour relies on the belief that an individual is part of a local community in which they need mutual help, support and love for one another [16, 17]. Therefore, an individual who practices prosocial behaviour that the community encourages will feel the sense of acceptance from his or her community group. It is because humans prefer giving help to the members of their group compared to strangers. Thus, the cultural difference can also cause some of the individuals having less tendency towards helping and putting their trust in strangers.

As the consequences, collective culture exists, which leads to egocentrism within a society. An egocentric society cares less for those who are outside of their group. This condition causes the antisocial behaviour and reduces the tendency of prosocial behaviour in the society. Fiedler et al. [18] argue about this situation where cultural differences can influence prosocial behaviour. *In-group favouritism* sees groups that share a similar identity as more straightforward to be helped compared to the out-group. According to Carlo and Randall [19], prosocial behaviour has two central concepts, which are the readiness to help and altruism.

Similarly, prosocial behaviour introduced by Penner et al. [20] through the development of *Prosocial Personality Battery* (PSB) to discuss two fundamental factor structures; *Other-oriented Empathy* and *Helpfulness*. The first factor; *Other-oriented Empathy* explains the cognitive and affective domain through the dimension of *social responsibility*, *mutual moral reasoning*, *other-oriented reasoning*, *empathic concern* and also *perspective taking*. Meanwhile, the second factor; *Helpfulness* relates to behavioural tendency through self-reported altruism and personal distress [3, 20–22].

Among the key aspects that have become the essence of focus in the discussion regarding prosocial behaviour are the causes and motives behind the formation of prosocial behaviour. The questions that arose through the discussion by Baron et al. [16], among others, to look at the motives, about how far an individual is involved in helping the needy and the situational and personal factors that cause the exposure of prosocial behaviour to a person. A low level of empathy as well as prosocial behaviour is said to contribute to the rejection of prosocial behaviour [17]. This condition shows that prosocial behaviour is linked to the voluntary actions to help others.

At the same time, individuals who provide the helping awareness are those with a high level of empathy. The present emotional, personal and situational influences are among the pulling factors of the existence of prosocial behaviour. The readiness to help among individuals largely depends on the existence of emotional effects, which involved the empathy aspect. When an individual possesses empathy, he or she will place him or herself in other people's shoes. Other people's misfortunes become the encouragement to the readiness to help among them. The help is as an effort to share emotions.

However, according to Carlo and Randall [19], a crowd situational factor makes an individual to have less tendency to behave prosocially. This condition shows that the sense of responsibility and readiness to help will decrease when they assume that other people can help. Each one hopes that there will be someone else who will help and take the responsibility. In today's globalisation challenges, this situation commonly occurs, which creates pluralistic ignorance when the crowd sees things that are unrelated to them. For example, the circumstances and mishaps within a society like wars, murders, robberies, deaths and missing persons received a cold shoulder and ignored on the social media. It is even more so if the circumstances befall on strangers. This scenario also leads to the news posts and shares on the social media that are lacking in empathy. Therefore, we must encourage the society, especially the Y generation to always behave prosocially in life. The dissemination of the caring and helpfulness culture within the identity of a society must be done especially concerning emergency circumstances. The society should be educated with awareness and with commitment in a good social environment to continue the prosocial behaviour.

Prosocial development is also associated with behaviourism and social learning theory [2] founded by Albert Bandura and his colleagues. Eisenberg et al. [2] argue using the social learning theory by presenting *internal cognitive* process as the critical role in behaviour influence. Therefore, impersonation is a critical process to achieve the socialisation standard of an individual's moral behaviour. Meanwhile, altruism is closely related to prosocial behaviour that can be described as an essential motive by voluntarily helping others without expecting anything in return [16, 20]. Altruism supports the prosocial concept as a motivational drive to unselfish behaviour to help others with sincerity and honesty. Therefore, an altruistic attitude is an attitude that prioritises the interests of others without expecting rewards in return.

From the aspect of readiness to help, the study of Carlo and Randall [19] states that compares to women, men are more fearless in offering help whether to those they know or strangers. The tendency to behave prosocially among men is higher from the aspect of exhibiting heroism, whereas women tend to help in the aspect of care, education and commitment. The arguments by Carlo and Randall [19] justify the different traits and characters between men and women. These gender differences produce different actions. Men tend to exhibit masculine actions such as daring to take the risk, being protective and having physical strength. On the contrary, women tend to exhibit more feminine actions such as loving and caring in giving a long-term commitment. Therefore, the gender differences resulted in different prosocial behaviours between men and women.

The studies on prosocial behaviour have also attracted the attention of the media scholars and researchers such as Gentile et al. [23], Wilson [24], Strasburger et al. [25] and Yates [26]. According to Wilson [23], if the media such as television and films expose children to the antisocial behaviours such as aggressiveness, then the same media should also be able to expose them to prosocial behaviour. Therefore, by giving instructions and controls especially to children regarding the choice of the media program, that should be able to help them become a more critical consumer towards the media content. It can encourage prosocial benefits from the time they spend in front of the television screen and other media devices such as films and the Internet.

Based on the previous studies, there were many studies on prosocial behaviours that are linked to media roles [24–27]. However, the group of people that the researchers often choose to be the subjects linked to prosocial behaviours are children and adolescent [23–25, 28, 29]. According to Dumova [27] based on social cognitive theory, children who are exposed to prosocial models and educational media content are more influenced by such prosocial behaviour during the interaction with their peers.

Strasburger et al. [25] state that researchers who are studying about prosocial learning through media often place the assumption where the media characters that portray traits such as kindness, mutual cooperation, responsible and unselfishness give the examples for children, especially for them to learn and imitate such behaviour. The study by Ostrov et al. [28] proves the existence of the link between media exposure and prosocial behaviour. In a longitudinal study conducted over 2 years, Ostrov et al. [28] examined the patterns and patents of change and development on the same sample that consisted of early kindergarten children, their parents and principals.

Ostrov et al. [28] study on the media exposure role is seen as for whether contributing to aggression as well as prosocial behaviour. The study on television programs as an interactive model contributes to positive learning through prosocial behaviour [26, 27]. Similarly, the television drama acts as 'facilitator' in forming prosocial behaviour [30]. Hence, in addition to having a link and relationship with violence and aggression affecting the behaviour of the audience, the television should also play its role in exposing the audience to prosocial behaviour. It can give benefits to the audience and the society.

The study by Udornpim and Singhal [31] highlights a character in a Japanese soap opera named 'Oshin' as a media role model among its audience in Thailand. In the outcomes of the study, Udornpim and Singhal [31] found that 'Oshin' presents a character who has traits such as perseverance, strong-willed and think positively as well as a willingness to help her family members who need aids. In the study, Udornpim and Singhal [31] have discussed 23 prosocial values, which among those are tolerance, independence, responsibility, mutual helpfulness, caring, forgiveness, gratefulness, diligence, high aspiration and love. The 'Oshin' character becomes a positive role model for the audience and illustrates how they could learn about prosocial values through the drama. Wallbank's [32] study also highlights the media model 'Robin Hood' in the discussion on the comparison between the antisocial and prosocial behaviour.

Meanwhile, Muller and Donnerstein [29] conducted two experimental studies on prosocial behaviour by screening an arousal film form and by using *the excitation transfer model.* The study by Muller and Donnerstein [29] on the subjects consisting of college students (male) aims to see the outcomes either from the aspect of positive and neutral behaviour. The subjects watched either the arousing erotic film or the controlled film that does not have the arousing erotic elements. The findings show that the *arousal* film can increase the subjects' punitive behaviour. Whereas, the subjects who watched the film that is absent from the arousing erotic elements show a more positive attitude [29]. Meanwhile, the correlation studies conducted by Gentile et al. [23] show a positive association between prosocial behaviour with *prosocial gaming exposure*.

The formation of prosocial behaviour is also associated with self-efficacy of individuals involved. Individual domination over self-efficacy can contribute to the differences in how he or she behaves. Carlo et al. [33] study measures prosocial behaviour based on social cognitive theory through the role of self-efficacy to prove the characteristics of the adolescent respondents in showing prosocial behaviour.

Carlo et al. [33] study found that there were differences in the types of prosocial behaviour among early and middle adolescents. Whereas, through the *prosocial agency* [34], humans can act as agents who set goals and behave following their personal and standard values that have been outlined based on their capability. It shows the contribution of self-efficacy and values to prosocial behaviour as discussed by Caprara and Steca [35].

4. Prosocial values and self-efficacy of religious society

The religious doctrine can be understood as a belief in God or magical and divine power such as deities [36, 37]. Preston et al. [37] and Hardy and Carlo [5] link religion to values and morals that exist within a society, while Saroglou et al. [6], as well as Norenzayan and Shariff [4], argue that religion is a part of a culture that set the values for people who practise religious life with prosocial standards. The definition of the concept of value depends on a few aspects, which originate from different fields such as political science, social sciences or religion. Whereas, Rokeach [38] sees the link between value with attitude and belief. The concept of value refers to the belief and attitude of an individual to translate it into a form of behaviour [38] whether the process produces something better or otherwise.

Whereas, the value from the Islamic point of view sees the relationship with Allah as the path of life in deciding [39], which includes ethical (*akhlak*) values (behaviour, beliefs and religion) and morality [40]. The appropriateness of every decision is based on the lifetime value that centres on the Islamic shariah. Syed Muhammad Naquib [39] also associates the concept of value with civility (*adab*). *Adab* in Islam centres on ethics, norms and morality.

Social and moral values are crucial as they are the root of well-being and harmony for a religious society. Noble values within a religion explain life that revolves around helping each other and living in peacefulness. Hence, religious prosociality values are in proximity with the noble values taught to a religious society [4]. There are studies on the prosocial behaviour that are viewed from the religious perspective, which becomes the catalyst for a high prosocial tendency within a society [4–6, 41]. Meanwhile, the study by Hardy and Carlo [5] proves that religiosity (the level of religious life) has a significant positive relationship with social behaviour predictor factors; kindness, compliant and altruistic values (prioritising other people's interests).

However, according to Malhotra [41], the link between religion and behaviour is closely related to the context of religious norms, especially for Christians who consider Sunday as the day to meet God. Therefore, most Christians behave more prosocially when the behaviour is linked to religious norms through religious importance on specific days (religious salience). The factor of religious belief is the driving force for a society to behave prosocially. According to Batara et al. [42], a society where its religious value is high is more willing to help others. Whereas, Sasaki et al. [43] argue that individuals with high religious value are better in their prosocial behaviour. However, according to Sasaki et al. [43], the religious influence on prosocial behaviour differs regarding an individual's acceptance. Even though religious factors contribute to prosocial behaviour, but undeniably there are other factors in the development of prosocial behaviour.

Prosocial behaviour is also aligned with the teachings of Islam that aim to encourage the society to practise noble values in life [44]. Islam as a religion that promotes peace and helpfulness accepts prosocial value as a decent value. It is because a religious society places a high emphasis on good religious values such as helpfulness, love and forgiveness. For Muslims, religion refers to Islam as *ad-deen* that can be explained as the submission to Allah as a way of life through the reinforcement of faith (*aqidah*) of the oneness of Allah, worships (*ibadah*), dealings (*muamalah*) and Islamic ethics (*akhlaq*).

In the same way with self-efficacy as a personal belief that influences an individual to behave in a certain way. According to Sania and Amena [45], self-efficacy has a significant association with religious belief. It means individuals who have self-efficacy awareness will be able to control better the actions and situations they meet. In the context of a society that holds onto a religious belief, self-efficacy fulfils the personal needs of an individual who believes and trusts in his or her capability. This belief leads to the ability and the faculty of the individual in assuming the responsibilities given unto him or her. The success in carrying out the responsibilities leads to outstanding human characteristics. A successful being is a balanced person between the physical and internal aspects of the self, which include self-confidence, goodwill and humbleness as well as consistently positive about success. However, according to Noornajihan [46], self-efficacy from the Islamic perspective is unlimited to only the belief that exists within the individual's self but also associated with the relationship with the Almighty Creator. Every Muslim believes in the oneness and the power of Allah as the Almighty Creator in the occurrence of everything.

5. Cognitive behaviour therapy: a psychological intervention influencing the formation of prosocial behaviour

Cognitive behavioural therapy (CBT) is a universal expression that originated from the cognitive model of affective disorders, which comprises of many approaches that are based on the postulation that cognition significantly influences emotion and behavioural impediment, and it also offers a wide range of evidence-based cognitive and behavioural techniques and therapies [7, 8]. Moghaddam and Dawson [8] added that despite the general assumption that cognition controls emotion and behaviour, the approaches in CBT have different emphasis, to name a few such as level of analysis (for example, situation-based versus person-based), levels of cognition (for example, prompt thoughts versus underlying central viewpoints) and problem-specificity (for instance, trans-diagnostic versus disorder-specific). Therefore, CBT involves a concerted effort between clients and therapists using a shared configuration to attain the treatment targets [7].

This concerted effort is idiographic in nature as it centres on customised therapy approach that best fits the patients' individual's conditions and needs. The customised intervention is built based on case formulation. According to Persons [9], case formulation is an empirically supported therapy (EST) in providing psychological treatment that is evidence-based that allows flexibility in addressing the patients' unique needs and also functions as guidelines for therapists in the decision-making process, especially in clinical treatment. Persons [9] further explained that an all-inclusive case formulation logically and coherently binds all of the following elements, which are (1) description of patient's symptoms, disorders and problems, (2) suggestion of hypotheses regarding the mechanisms that cause the disorders and problems and (3) suggestion of the latest outcomes of the present disorders and problems as well as the roots of the mechanisms. In cognitive behavioural therapy, a therapist begins a case formulation by obtaining a diagnosis through the collection of assessment facts. He or she then structures the diagnosis into the individualised formulation of the case and uses it to facilitate the task of designing a therapeutic strategy. Patient's consent is necessary before the treatment begins, and once it starts, the formulation will serve as decision-making guidelines for the therapist. This collaborative treatment enables the therapist to collect critical data in observing the treatment progress. It also allows the therapist to make the necessary adjustment [9].

Negative social exchanges refer to the unwelcome and unsympathetic exchanges among members of a social network [47]. The examples of the negative social exchanges are neglect, rejection, insensitivity, interference and unwanted advice (Brooks and Dunkel Schetter, 2011; Newsom et al., 2005; Rook, 1998 in Silva et al., 2016 [47]). It is an ironic social exchange where members of a social network assume that they are behaving helpfully, but in the actual sense, they are not (Oku and Keith, 1998 in Silva et al., 2016 [47]). Research indicates that negative social exchange negatively influences health [47], therefore about self-efficacy and development of prosocial behaviour, the negative social exchange could pose a threat in promoting higher level self-efficacy among people with low of self-efficacy and behaving antisocially.

6. Conclusions

The concept of self-efficacy explains the attitude of individuals who believe in themselves. It becomes the catalyst for the rational cognitive process in shaping the behaviour of an individual. Hence, self-efficacy that is inherent in each person can shape a reasonable and mature prosocial value in a society. If a society has a high self-efficacy, then the condition of the society to change to a better state is also high. There is, however, a challenge in having positive-minded individuals with high self-efficacy. In dealing with the reality of life, humans are often tested with different trials and tribulations whether they are personal, family, academic or workplace problems. People with good self-efficacy accept the trials and tribulations as a challenge. However, if an individual accepts the pitfalls negatively, then they will not put efforts to overcome them. Even more so, they will see the problems as difficulties that decrease their motivation.

Academic scholars often relate the relationship between the level of self-efficacy with positivism that contributes to the formation of individuals' prosocial behaviour. Individuals who have a decent self-efficacy level will see the world with utmost positivism. They can translate such positivism through the proper behaviour that is inherent in themselves. They have positive ways of thinking that project a fair view among those who are around them. Thus, the readiness to help and love for each other exists as the essential elements in prosocial behaviour.

This condition is also associated with the role of religion that encourages its society to practice tolerance and kindness to others. A society that is educated with positive actions such as being helpful with one another, loving as well as having an emphatic soul, interacts easier within a peaceful and harmonious atmosphere. A society that has a prosocial personality tends to behave positively more easily. Therefore, the efforts to help based on the concern towards other people become the motivational factor that is closely associated with prosocial behaviour. Prosocial behaviour is a positive behaviour that can contribute towards better societal change. A decent societal community is those who are complementing each other, living peacefully without disagreement as well as respecting different views among them. All the religions in this world promote peace and safety, which supports prosocial value. The attitudes such as helpfulness, respect and love are the requisite of religious society that leads towards the reinforcement of prosocial behaviour through self-efficacy.

Thus, having the data of patient's negative social exchanges at the start of the treatment allows a therapist to customise the intervention through the formation of a precise and unique psychological intervention that is sensitive towards the patient's most fragile areas and the ones that need to be addressed promptly. This idiographic customisation allows a better understanding of the kind of negative social exchanges that could hinder the attainment of a higher level of self-efficacy. The recognition will help the therapist to strategically facilitate the alteration of the patient's thought process into becoming more harmonious, which resulted in better self-efficacy level that later helps an individual behaves more prosocially.

Acknowledgements

This research was funded by Universiti Kebangsaan Malaysia (UKM) through Research Grant University (GUP-2018-011).

Conflict of interest

I have no conflict of interest and yes I have read and understood the guidelines on copyright.

Author details

Rosmawati Mohamad Rasit* and Siti Zuhrah Che Ab Razab
Universiti Kebangsaan Malaysia, Bangi, Selangor, Malaysia

*Address all correspondence to: rosmawati@ukm.edu.my

References

[1] Bandura A. Self-efficacy: Toward a unifying theory of behavioral change. Psychology Review. 1977;**84**(2):191-215

[2] Eisenberg N, Fabes RA, Spinrad Tracy L. Prosocial development. In: Damon W, Lerner RM, Eisenberg N, editors. Handbook of Child Psychology Social, Emotional dan Personality Development. 6th ed. New Jersey: John Wiley and Sons, Inc; 2006. pp. 646-718

[3] Penner LA, Dovidio JF, Piliavin JA, Schroeder DA. Prosocial behavior: Multilevel perspectives. Annual Review of Psychology. 2005;**56**(14):14.1-14.28

[4] Norenzayan A, Shariff AF. The origin and evolution of religious prosociality. Science. 2008;**322**(5898):58-62

[5] Hardy SA, Carlo G. Religiosity and prosocial behaviours in adolescence: The mediating role of prosocial values. Journal of Moral Education. 2005;**34**(2):231-249

[6] Saroglou V, Pichon I, Trompette L, Verschueren M, Dernelle R. Prosocial behavior and religion: New evidence based on projective measures and peer ratings. Journal for the Scientific Study of Religion. 2005;**44**(3):323-348

[7] National Collaborating Centre for Mental Health. Alcohol-Use Disorders: The NICE Guideline on Diagnosis, Assessment and Management of Harmful Drinking and Alcohol Dependence. British Psychological Society and The Royal College of Psychiatrists; 2011. 612 p. ISBN: 978-1-904671-26-8. Available from: https://www.ncbi.nlm.nih.gov/books/n/nicecg115/pdf/

[8] Moghaddam, NG. and Dawson, DL. Cognitive-behavioural therapy. In: Formulation in Action: Applying Psychological Theory to Clinical Practice. UK: De Gruyter; 2016. p. 35-39. DOI: 10.1515/9783110471014-006

[9] Persons JB. The Case Formulation Approach to Cognitive-Behavior Therapy. New York: Guilford Publications; 2008

[10] Bandura A. Social Foundations of Thought and Action: A Social Cognitive Theory. New Jersey: Prentice-Hall; 1986

[11] Bandura A. Self-efficacy. In: Ramachaudran VS, editor. Encyclopedia of Human Behavior. Vol. 4. New York: Academic Press; 1994. pp. 71-81. Available from: http://www.des.emory.edu/mfp/BanEncy.html

[12] Bandura A. Social cognitive theory. In: Vasta R, editor. Annals of Child Development. Vol. 6. Greenwich, CT: JAI Press; 1989. pp. 1-60

[13] Awais M, Qurat-ul-Ain. Relationship between self-efficacy a type personality and leader effectiveness. International Journal of Engineeering Research and Management. 2018;**5**(1):33-38

[14] Eklund J, Loeb C, Hansen EM, Anderson-Wallin AC. Who cares about others? Empathic self-efficacy as an antecedents to pro-social behaviour. Current Research in Social Psychology. 2012;**20**:31-41. Available from: https://uiowa.edu/crisp/sites/uiowa.edu.crisp/files/20.3.pdf

[15] Hastings PD, Utendale WT, Sullivan C. The socialization of prososial development. In: Grusec JE, Hastings PD, editors. Handbook of Socialization: Theory and Research. New York: Guilford Publications; 2007. pp. 638-661

[16] Baron RA, Branscombe NR, Byrne D. Social Psychology. 12th ed. USA: Pearson Education; 2009

[17] Twenge JM, Ciarocco NJ, Baumeister RF, Nathan DeWall C, Bartels JM. Social exclusion decreases prosocial behavior. Journal of

Personality and Social Psychology. 2007;**92**(1):56-66

[18] Fiedler S, Hellman DM, Dorrough AR, Glockner A. Cross-national in-group favoritism in prosocial behavior: Evidence from Latin and North America. Judgment and Decision making. 2018;**13**(1):42060

[19] Carlo G, dan Randall BA. The development of a measure of prosocial behaviors for late adolescents. Journal of Youth and Adolescence. 2002;**31**(1):31-44

[20] Penner LA, Fritzsche BA, Craiger JP, Freifeld TR. Measuring the prosocial personality. In: Butcher J, Spielberger CD, editors. Advances in Personality Assessment. Vol. 10. Hillsdale, New Jersey: Erlbaum; 1995. pp. 147-164

[21] Gillath O, Karantzas G. Predicting prosocial personality from attachment facets: Are some facets more critical than others? In: Prosiding Generations of Relationships and Relationships accross Generations Conference. 2007. pp. 41-52

[22] Finkelstein MA, Penner LA, Brannick MT. Motive, role identity and prosocial personality as predictors of volunteer activity. Social Behavior and Personality. 2005;**33**(4):403-418

[23] Gentile DA, Anderson CA, Yukawa S, Ihori N, Saleem M, Ming LK, et al. The effects of prosocial video games on prosocial behaviors: International evidence from correlational, longitudinal and experimental studies. Personality and Social Psychology Bulletin. 2009;**35**(6):752-763

[24] Wilson BJ. Media and children's aggression, fear and altruism. Journal of Children and Media. 2008;**18**(1):87-118

[25] Strasburger VC, Wilson BJ, Jordan AB. Prosocial effects of media. In: Children, Adolescents and the Media. 2th ed. Thousand Oaks, CA: Sage Publications, Inc; 2009. pp. 117-144. Available from: http://people.oregonstate.edu/~flayb/MY%20COURSES/H549%20Mass%20Media%20and%20Health%20%20Winter%202012/Readings/Strasburger%20etal09%20Ch_4%20Prosocial%20effects%20of%20media.pdf

[26] Yates BL. Modeling strategies for prosocial television: A review. In: Kertas Kerja Dibentangkan di Open Paper Competition AEJMC Siutheast Colloqium; 4-6 Mac. Lexington, Kentucky. 1999

[27] Dumova T. Prosocial learning. International Journal of Learning. 2006;**2**(9):183-194. Available from: http://www.learning-journal.com

[28] Ostrov JM, Gentile DA, Crick NR. Media exposure, aggression and prosocial behaviour during early childhood: A longitudinal study. Social Development. 2006;**15**:612-627

[29] Muller CW, Donnerstein E. Film-facilitated arousal and prosocial behavior. Journal of Experimental Social Psychology. 1981;**17**:31-41

[30] Baran SJ, Chase LJ, Courtright JA. Television drama as a facilitator of prosocial behavior: "The Waltons". Journal of Broadcasting. 1979;**23**(3):277-284

[31] Udornpim K, Singhal A. Oshin, a pro-social media role model, in Thailand. Keio Communication Review. 1999;(21):3-21

[32] Wallbank J. Antisocial and prosocial behavior among contemporary Robon hoods. Personality and Individual Differences. 1985;**6**(1):11-19

[33] Carlo G, Hausmann A, Christiansen S, Randall BA. Sociocognitive and behavioral correlates of a measure of

prosocial tendencies for adolescent. Journal of Early Adolescence. 2003;**23**(1):107-134

[34] Bandura A. The evolution of social cognitive theory. In: Smith KG, Hitt MA, editors. Great Minds in Management. Oxford: Oxford University Press; 2005. pp. 9-35. Available from: http://www.des.emory.edu/mfp/Bandura2005.pdf

[35] Caprara GV, Steca P. Prosocial agency: The contribution of values and self-efficacy beliefs to prosocial behavior across ages. Journal of Social and Clinical Psychology. 2007;**26**(2):218-239

[36] Macionis JJ, Plummer K. Sociology a Global Introduction. 3th ed. Harlow: Pearson Education Limited; 2005

[37] Preston JL, Ritter RS, Hernandez JI. Principles of religious prosociality: A review and reformulation. Social and Personality Psychology Compass. 2010;**4**(8):574-590

[38] Rokeach M. The Nature of Human Values. New York: The Free Press; 1973

[39] Syed Muhammad Naquib A. Prolegomena to the Metaphysics of Islam: An Exposition of the Fundamental Elements of the Worldview of Islam. Kuala Lumpur: International Institute of Islamic Thought and Civilization; 1995

[40] Sawai RP, Abdullah S, Baharudin DF, Ismail N. Penerapan nilai-nilai Islam melalui penggunaan media dalam pendidikan. In: Mustafa MZ, Rahim AM, Ahmad ZA, Ramle NA, editors. Representasi Islam dalam Media. Nilai: Universiti Sains Islam Malaysia; 2011. pp. 53-61

[41] Malhotra D. (When) are religious people nicer? Religious salience and the “Sunday effect” on pro-social behavior. Judgment and Decision making. 2010;**5**(5):138-143. Available from: http://journal.sjdm.org/10/10216/jdm10216.html

[42] Batara JBL, Franco PS, Quiachon MAM, Sembrero d, Dianelle Rose M. Effects of religious priming concepts on prosocial behavior towards ingroup and outgroup. Europe’s Journal of Psychology. 2016;**12**(4):635-644

[43] Sasaki JY, Kim H, Mojaverian T, Kelly LDS, Park IY, Janusonis S. Religion priming differentially increases prososial behavior among variants of dopamine D4 receptor (DRD4) genre. Social Cognitive and Affective Neuroscience. 2013;**8**:209-215

[44] Mohamad Rasit R. Structural equation modelling (SEM) analysis of influence of religious films on pro-social behaviour of audience. Asian Social Science. 2015;**11**(18):42-48

[45] Shah SS, Zehra AA. Religious faith, flourishing and self-efficacy in young adults: A correlational study. Global Journal of Arts, Humanities and Social Sciences. 2015;**3**(10):34-45

[46] Noornajihan J. Efikasi Kendiri: Perbandingan antara Islam dan Barat. Global Journal Al-Thaqafah. 2014;**4**(2):89-98

[47] Silva NM, Henrie JA, Patrick JH. Personality, negative social exchanges, and physical health among bereaved adults. Health Psychology Open. 2016;(1):-14. DOI: 10.1177/2055102916637877

Section 2

Psychological Applications of CBT

Chapter 4

A Distorted Body Image: Cognitive Behavioral Therapy for Body Dysmorphic Disorder

Norzihan Ayub, Patricia Joseph Kimong and Guan Teik Ee

Abstract

Body dysmorphic disorder (BDD) is one of the mental disorders that warrant more research due to the current challenges and complexity of human life. A search through Medline, Academic Search Premier, PsycINFO, and PsyArticles, using "body dysmorphic disorder" and "intervention" keywords, showed that a total of 186 articles had been published for the past 25 years. BDD was added to the obsessive-compulsive and related disorder spectrum in the *Diagnostic and Statistical Manual of Mental Disorder-5* (2013). BDD is a preoccupation with an imagined defect in physical appearance by individual who looks normal which causes low self-esteem and co-morbids with other mental health problems. Individuals with BDD often end up with dermatological treatment and cosmetic surgery. However, in most cases, they frequently experience a dissatisfaction with the results and worsen the individual condition. Therefore, psychological intervention is needed to treat individuals with BDD to combat their negative perceptions on physical appearance. Research has shown that one of the effective interventions in treating individuals with BDD is cognitive behavioral therapy (CBT). Some techniques that are recommended are psychoeducation, restructuring cognitive, exposure and ritual prevention, and others. This paper aims to discuss the clinical diagnosis and CBT intervention as a treatment for individual with BDD.

Keywords: body dysmorphic disorder, cognitive behavioral therapy, body image, skin picking, obsessive-compulsive disorder

1. Introduction

Body image is one of the first individual characteristics noticed by others and has an important impact on self-image and social interactions. Research study revealed that there is a relationship between self-esteem and body dissatisfaction. This proves that beauty has a connection with self-esteem and self-image [1].

Body image is not just a cognitive construct but also a reflection of attitude and interaction with others. Being concerned and worried about the appearance and body image is normal and common among many people, mostly in female. However, if the individual is overly worried and concerned and affects a person's functionality, then it is considered a problem and pathological.

Body image encompasses perceptions, thoughts, and feelings about the body that are influenced by development, perception, and sociocultural factors [2]. In some people, perception has been shaped in such a way that it contradicts with reality. One of the most common forms of this disorder is body dysmorphic disorder (BDD). BDD is a severe disorder defined by a preoccupation with perceived imperfections in appearance and resulting in repetitive behaviors, which also causes a clinically significant distress or functional impairment [3]. BDD also has a high rate of suicidality [4, 5]. BDD typically begins during early adolescence and appears to be common in adults. BDD, previously known as dysmorphobia, represents a psychotic delusional state, whereby the individual was unable to realize, even for a fleeting moment, that their ideas were irrational. Individuals with BDD believe they looked ugly or unattractive when in reality they look normal and attractive. Many people with BDD will seek unnecessary dermatologic, dental, and other cosmetic treatments in hopes of removing their negative perceptions on physical appearance. These procedures have poor outcomes and lead to individuals distress, often worsening the symptoms and leading to the dissatisfaction and loss of self-esteem [6]. Feelings of frustration, hopelessness, or shame resulting from engagement in or disturbance of rituals can also lead to anger outbursts and may involve physical aggression [7].

2. Diagnosis and clinical assessment of body dysmorphic disorder

Previously, BDD was considered a somatoform disorder because its central feature is a psychological preoccupation with somatic issues. However, increasing evidence has indicated it was more closely related to obsessive-compulsive disorder (OCD), accounting for its relocation to the obsessive-compulsive and related disorders section in the *Diagnostic and Statistical Manual of Mental Disorders-5* [3]. The diagnostic criteria of BDD are as follows:

2.1 Appearance preoccupation

Individuals with BDD are constantly preoccupied and persistently complaining about their appearance which they deem horrible and intrusive [8]. Individuals with BDD exhibit perfectionistic thinking and maladaptive attractiveness beliefs [9]. The average number of body areas that is of a concern to these individuals was five to seven, and preoccupation may focus on any areas of the body and commonly involves the face, nose, hair, skin, breast, teeth, and others [3]. However, some can concern only one area. Concerns range from looking unattractive to looking disgusting. These thoughts are very distressing and are associated with a feeling of low self-esteem, rejection sensitivity, embarrassment, and shame [10]. Generally, they spend at least an hour a day of thinking about the supposed appearance flaws. On average, they will spend between 3 and 8 hours a day on this [10]. Some individuals are also concerned about the perceived asymmetry of body areas. A study showed that females with BDD were more likely to be preoccupied with their hips, weight, breasts, legs, pick their skin and disguise with makeup, while males with BDD were more likely to be preoccupied with their body build, genitals, and hair thinning [11, 12]. Muscle dysmorphia, a form of BDD occurring mostly in male individuals, consists of preoccupation with the idea that one's body is too small or insufficiently lean or insufficiently muscular. In reality, these individuals actually have a normal-looking body and are muscular. Some are also very preoccupied with other areas such as their hair and skin. A majority of them also practices diet and exercise extremely that in turn leads to bodily damage [3].

2.2 Ritual

Individuals with BDD also perform ritual behavior by mirror checking or compensating in attempts to alleviate their concerns and anxiety. Excessive grooming, camouflaging, and skin picking are also common in BDD [8, 13]. Some individuals are excessively tan, for example, to darken "pale" skin or diminish perceived acne. In addition, some individuals repeatedly change their clothes such as to camouflage the perceived defects, or some individuals compulsively shop for their beauty products [3]. Many of these behaviors are considered compulsive, in that they are repetitive and difficult to resist or control the rituals.

2.3 Distress or impairment in social, occupational, or other important areas of functioning

People with BDD also have the idea of reference which means they think everything that goes on in their world is related to them. This thinking and perception can cause disruption in their lives. Impairment in functioning can include problems with any aspect of social functioning that is caused by BDD, such as problems with relationships, socializing, intimacy, or difficulty being around other people. It also includes problems with the ability to function in a job, academically, or in one's role in life [14].

Among adults, BDD results in high rates of occupational impairment, unemployment, social dysfunction, and social isolation [15]. Similarly, BDD in youths is associated with major functional impairment, including reduced academic performance, social withdrawal, and dropping out of school [16]. They may even become housebound [8]. Overall, individuals with BDD have a markedly poor quality of life.

2.4 Other features of BDD

2.4.1 Avoidance behaviors

Individuals with BDD also avoid some social situations because they feel ashamed and embarrassed about their appearance. They are also concerned and worried about how people perceive their appearance. They always assume and think that people are laughing and talking about them because of how they look. They avoid social gatherings, interaction with friends, dating, or places where their body can be seen or exposed such as parties, events, schooling environment, or crowded places such as shopping malls [17]. They think that everyone thinks they are unattractive, and because of that, they avoid any social or leisure activities. In one study, 18% had dropped out of school primarily due to BDD [18], and in another study, 22% had dropped out of school due to BDD [15].

2.4.2 Delusional beliefs

Individual with BDD also have delusional beliefs. They do not recognize that the appearance flaws they perceive are nonexistent [19]. They also tend to think that most people share their views of the supposed defects. People with delusional beliefs also realize that their appearance has a psychological cause; they simply think their beliefs are true [17]. Individuals with BDD display delusion beliefs, believing that people around them notice their defect and evaluate them negatively as a consequence of their ugliness.

Individuals with BDD who have delusional beliefs are also difficult to treat. Research done by other researchers has shown that 79% of patients have had ideas or delusions of reference, believing that others take special notice of the perceived defects [15, 18].

2.4.3 Skin picking

Individuals with BDD also compulsively pick their skin to try to remove any imperfections in their body. They may use their fingers or other tools such as needles, knives, razors, pins, and other sharp objects that can harm their skin. This ritualistic behavior can take hours a day and can cause tissue damage. However, they have no intention of damaging their skin, but they have difficulties in trying to control the ritualistic behavior [17].

3. Body dysmorphic disorder and other mental illnesses

Individual who meet the diagnostic criteria for BDD will often also develop other mental illnesses. BDD is also associated with eating disorder, anxiety disorder, major depression disorder (MDD), substance use disorder, social phobia, obsessive-compulsive disorder (OCD), panic disorder, and post-traumatic stress disorder [8, 10, 20, 21]. Among BDD sufferers, 94% reported that they felt depressed at some point due to their illness [10]. In the largest comorbidity study (n = 293), the most common disorders were MDD (lifetime prevalence of 76%), social anxiety disorder (37%), and OCD (32%) [21].

OCD and social phobia have also been found to have a high lifetime prevalence in BDD individual of 32–33% and 37–39%, respectively. About 10–15% of those with BDD have a lifetime history of anorexia nervosa or bulimia nervosa. Moreover, 2–7% of BDD have a history of somatoform disorder [8, 21, 22].

Meanwhile, 60% of subjects in one study reported that their substance use began after symptoms of BDD and 68% reported that their illness contributed to their substance use becoming problematic [23, 24]. Among individual with BDD, 42.6% reported an alcohol use disorder, and 30.1% reported a cannabis use disorder [23, 24]. Muscle dysmorphia, a specific type of BDD, was also found to have the highest rates of substance abuse such as street drugs and alcohol at the rate of 86% [10]. Moreover, 68% of individuals with a lifetime substance use disorder reported that BDD contributed to their substance use disorder [23]. On the other hand, studies suggest that certain psychoactive drugs, such as cocaine or methamphetamine, may worsen obsession symptoms [25].

Besides the comorbidity, BDD is also associated with increased suicidal ideation. The extant literature suggests a particularly strong link between BDD and elevated rates of suicidal thoughts and suicidal behaviors. Up to 75% of individuals with BDD report experiencing lifetime suicidal ideation, and 25% of individual with BDD report a history of making a suicide attempt. The data suggest a rate of completed suicide up to 45 times that of the general population [26]. The delusional variant of BDD is considered more severe and leads to suicide [27, 28]. BDD appears to engender the four psychological constructs thought to predict suicide: perceived burdensomeness, thwarted belongingness, low fear of death, and high physical pain tolerance [29].

The other researcher also stated that physically painful BDD behaviors that involved cosmetic surgery and restrictive eating would be associated with suicide attempts but not suicide-related ideation because these behaviors increase capability for, but not thoughts about, suicide [29].

4. Cognitive behavioral model for understanding body dysmorphic disorder (BDD)

Few researchers have contributed to a cognitive behavioral model for understanding BDD [30, 31]. According to this model, an individual's behavior and emotions are thought to be determined by their interpretation of events. It is not the incidents or events that determine what the individual feels but of how he or she perceives it. However, many people always accept their perceptions of situations or events as true and may even be unaware that they are making these negative interpretations because this happens automatically to them [17].

According to Beck, the foundation of cognitive behavioral is that individuals develop an understanding about themselves, other people, and their personal worlds. Core beliefs are central ideas about the self and others [32]. Individuals with BDD usually have negative core beliefs relating to their personal worthwhile underlying their negative view of appearance [17]. They always overestimate the meaning and importance of perceived imperfections and misinterpret them as major personal flaws. An example of core beliefs about themselves is "If I am ugly, everyone will not love me and I will be isolated" or "I am worthless." They interpret minor imperfections in appearance as a signal of major flaws because they hold predisposed beliefs they learned previously [17].

Besides having personal negative core beliefs about themselves, individual with BDD always has a negative core belief about others around them such as thinking "people only like sexy body." This leads to their core beliefs and assumptions that they are unattractive and worthless. They tend to jump to conclusions without considering any explanations for their negative interpretation of situations [17]. Perceived imperfections of their negative interpretations will lead to negative emotions, such as anxiety, shame, and sadness, which further increase selective attention to perceived flaws.

As a way of reducing their anxiety, shame, or sadness, individuals with BDD will engage in ritual behavior or avoidance of social situations. Avoidance behavior includes avoiding social contact and other situations such as going to school or parties. Meanwhile, ritual behaviors include mirror checking, skin picking, reassurance seeking, repeated plastic surgery, and excessive grooming situations [17]. Since the rituals and avoidance behaviors can temporarily reduce negative emotions, they are negatively reinforced and, in this way, are hypothesized to maintain dysfunctional BDD-related beliefs. Therefore, cognitive behavioral therapy (CBT) for BDD targets cognitive, emotional, and behavioral factors and generally includes psychoeducation, cognitive intervention, exposure to avoided situations, and prevention of rituals and perceptual retraining such as to reduce selective attention to details such as appearance flaws [33].

The model of BDD from the other researcher focuses on the experience of people with BDD when they are alone [34]. The model begins with the trigger of an external representation of the individual's body image, typically in front of a mirror. The process of selective attention begins by focusing on specific aspects of the external representation, which leads to a heightened awareness and relative exaggeration of certain features. As a result of this process, the person with BDD constructs a distorted mental representation of their body image. Mirror gazing activates idealized values about the importance of appearance and, in some individual with BDD, values about perfectionism or symmetry and thinking of the self as an esthetic object. This leads to a negative esthetic appraisal and comparisons of three different images—the external representation (usually in a mirror), the ideal body image, and the distorted body image. These repeated comparisons leave them uncertain about their appearance, which encourages for further mirror gazing. The individual with BDD desire to see exactly how he or she looks is only rewarded by looking in the mirror. However, the longer the person looks, the worse they feel and the more the belief of ugliness and unattractiveness is reinforced. When not looking in a mirror, the individual may focus and give more attention to his or her internal body image and ruminate on its ugliness. There is often a marked discrepancy between the actual and the ideal body images, and this inevitably leads to a depressed mood and negative thoughts [34].

5. The development of body dysmorphic disorder

An understanding of how BDD develops is still uncertain, and studies about this are still restricted compared to other disorders. However, there are several key factors that play a role in the development of BDD such as serotonin hypothesis and other neurotransmitters, abnormalities in the brain, culture and mass media roles, parenting styles, environment, and genetic predispositions that contribute to BDD.

5.1 The serotonin hypothesis and other neurotransmitters

Individuals with BDD may have imbalance in the brain's chemical serotonin. In support of this theory, BDD often improves with serotonin reuptake inhibitor medications, which help to boost serotonin in the brain to a healthy level. The brain consists of billions of nerve cells and serotonin. Serotonin, one of the neurotransmitters, is a natural brain chemical that carries information from nerve cell to nerve cell. Serotonin permits cells to communicate with one another and to function [10].

Serotonin is especially abundant in certain parts of the brain that may be especially important in BDD. It is critical to many bodily functions including mood, memory, cognition, appetite, eating behavior, sleep, sexual behavior, and pain. It restrains aggressive and destructive behaviors. Serotonin is involved in a variety of disorders such as OCD and depression. Serotonin is also involved in the visual system and visual processing, and it may help protect animals from overreacting to unimportant sensory input from the environment. This is interesting given that people with BDD appear to overfocus on unimportant details of appearance and "overreact" to nonexistent threats. Serotonin reuptake inhibitor medication helps people become less "overreactive" and less focused on minor appearance flaws. In addition to possible effects on the visual system, serotonin reuptake inhibitors might alleviate BDD symptoms by increasing serotonin release in the striatum and other key brain areas and by inhibiting an overactive amygdala [10]. It is likely that other neurotransmitters are also involved in BDD. For example, dopamine, which may, in combination with serotonin, be particularly important in the development delusional form of BDD [10].

5.2 Abnormalities in the brain

BDD highly likely involves a complex interplay of dysfunction in several neural regions and systems of the brain. Left-sided prefrontal and temporal regions involved in visual processing of faces, and amygdala hyperreactivity, may play a role in development of BDD [10]. Dysfunction in frontal-striatal brain circuits may also be involved. A study conducted by researchers which compared women with BDD to healthy women without BDD using MRI scans to visualize the brain's structure. The researchers found that the BDD group's MRI scans differed in subtle ways from healthy woman. There were differences in the caudate, a C-shaped structure deep in the brain's core (the striatum), which regulates voluntary movements, habits, learning, and cognitions and may be linked to repetitive or ritual behaviors in BDD [10].

Other brain regions might also be involved in BDD. A small neuroimaging study that used single photon emission computed tomography (SPECT) showed various areas of hyperactivation in diffused areas of the brain such as the frontal, temporal, occipital, and parietal lobes [10]. Possible that all of these areas may be involved, it makes sense that the fusiform face and extrastriate body areas, in particular, which are located in the temporal/occipital area, are important in the perception of the body image, and facial emotion perception might play a role. Damage to these areas as well as the parietal lobe can impair perception of bodies and faces [10].

Moreover, one study from the Department of Psychiatry and Biobehavioral Sciences, which studied the abnormalities of visual processing and frontostriatal systems in body dysmorphic disorder, found out that individuals with BDD also demonstrated visual processing and frontostriatal abnormalities when viewing their own face. Moreover, brain activity in these systems correlates with symptom severity. The frontostriatal system findings, especially *orbitofrontal cortex* (OFC) and caudate hyperactivity, suggest possible similar neural pathophysiology to obsessive–compulsive disorder. Abnormalities in visual processing systems may contribute distorted perceptual input to frontostriatal systems, which may be associated with the experience of aversion and that may subsequently mediate obsessive thought patterns and urges to perform compulsive behaviors [35].

A study also discovers that orbitofrontal cortex and anterior cingulate cortex volumes of individual with BDD were significantly smaller than healthy individuals. The individual with BDD brain has more white substances than the healthy individuals [10, 36]. There is also a tendency of an increase of thalamic volume in individual with BDD compared with healthy individual. Evidence also found that right amygdala volume has shown a significant correlation with BDD symptom severity, which suggests a different lateral involvement of the brain regions [37].

5.3 Genetic

There have been small studies investigating genetic factors underlying BDD. Nevertheless, heredity and genetic factors do appear to contribute to BDD. Having certain genes will increase the chances of having certain personality traits, where certain brain circuits are hyperreactive and other characteristics may further increase the risk of getting BDD. Research studies also found that about 20% of people with BDD have at least one first-degree relative such as parent, sibling, or child with BDD. About 6% of all first-degree relatives have BDD. This rate is an estimated three to six times higher than in the general population [10]. BDD probably runs in families because family members share genes that increase the risk of getting BDD. In addition, a preliminary genetics study by researchers found that a certain form of a gene called the GABAA-γ2 receptor gene was more common in people with BDD than in those without BDD [10].

Moreover, 8% of individuals with BDD have a family member also diagnosed with BDD, a statistic four to eight times prevalent in the general population [38]. Some studies show that BDD is more common in individual whose blood relatives also have this condition or obsessive-compulsive disorder [39]. The association between body dysmorphic symptoms and obsessive-compulsive symptoms is largely explained by shared genetic factors. Environmental risk factors were largely unique to each phenotype. These results also support current recommendations to group BDD together with OCD in the same *DSM-5*, although comparison with other phenotypes such as somatoform disorders and social phobia is needed [39].

In addition, the results of twin studies indicate that genetic factors account for approximately 42–44% of the variance in BDD-like symptoms, with the remaining variance being account for by non-shared environmental influences [40, 41].

A twin study in females that operate self-report measures of dysmorphic concerns and concerns about body odor and body malfunction from the United Kingdom twin registry found that genetic factors accounted for approximately 44% of the variance of dysmorphic concerns [40].

5.4 Cultural factors

There are studies that have examined the role of culture in the development of BDD. The tendency to link body attractiveness with positive personal qualities has become a cultural stereotype in the world. Because of the stereotype, people start to be concerned and anxious about their looks and appearance although they are normal with no defects. They exaggerated worry about what other people say about their appearance.

BDD is not specific to one country or culture. Furthermore, cases of BDD have been reported in a variety of countries, including the United States, Canada, Europe, China, Japan, and Africa [27, 42–44]. In Japan, for example, it is called shubo kyofu. Shubo kyofu is characterized by excessive fear of having bodily deformity, and it is similar with BDD. According to the traditional Japanese diagnostic system, shubo kyofu is a subtype of taijin kyofusho (social anxiety), a cultural syndrome characterized by fear and avoidance of interpersonal relationship [45].

In Korea, females typically more prefer slim and skinny bodies. Even though they are normal or underweight, they strive for weight control routinely. Severely losing weight for women has become a social problem due to the appearance-oriented trend in Japan. A study conducted by researchers from the Department of Dental Hygiene, Kangwon University, was performed by 200 health-related and 200 health-unrelated college students, respectively, at K College in Gangwon province. The study showed that as a result of analyzing the relationship between the BMI of the female students and their dissatisfied parts of the body, overweight female students were more dissatisfied with the entire lower parts of their body and whole body, and the female students of normal weight were more dissatisfied with their waist and belly than the other groups. The underweight female students were more dissatisfied with their chests and breasts. But there were no differences in the way they wanted to try and change dissatisfied parts of the body [46].

Meanwhile, a group of researchers from Brazil did a study in Abdominal Plastic Surgery Unit of the São Paulo Hospital, Brazil. A high prevalence of BDD symptoms was found among candidates for abdominoplasty and body weight, and shape concerns were significantly associated with severity of BDD symptoms. It was found that the more severe the symptoms of BDD, the higher the level of concern with body weight and shape. Individuals with BDD having distorted self-perception of body shape or distorted comparative perception of body image were, respectively, 3.67 or 5.93 times more likely to show more severe symptoms of BDD than individual with a more accurate perception [47].

To the best of our knowledge, there has not been any published literature on the prevalence of BDD among patients in an Asian population. However, the results coming from the researchers in Singapore hospitals show that BDD is quite prevalent among patients who have received cosmetic rhinoplasty. BDD patients are likely to have poorer subjective outcomes after surgery although they may experience some improvement in satisfaction when compared to before surgery [48].

One study has conducted the only cross-cultural study published to date and found that BDD prevalence rates in BDD are fairly similar between American (N = 101, 4%) and German students (N = 133, 5.3%) [49]. Cultural factors may play a role in which body parts are of a concern and how other BDD symptoms are expressed, as different cultures may have variations in esthetic standards of beauty, but this has yet to be studied in relation to BDD [50].

It appears that cultural values and preferences may influence and shape BDD symptoms to some degree. For example, eyelid concerns appear common in Japan but rare in Western countries. Worried about displeasing other people by being unattractive also seems more common in Japan than in the United States. Some people say that their BDD symptoms began when they moved to another culture and felt that they looked different and did not fit in [10].

5.5 Environment and life experiences

Environment and life experiences may contribute to BDD, especially if they involve negative social evaluations about someone's appearance, body or self-image, or even childhood neglect or abuse. Bullying has been shown to be associated with BDD, and most episodes were interpersonal and occurred during grade school or middle school [51]. BDD symptoms were higher when adolescents self-reported more appearance teasing and higher social anxiety. Moreover, it was appearance teasing by cross-sex peers, rather than same-sex peers, that was uniquely associated with elevated BDD symptoms [52]. In longitudinal studies of environmental risk factors in BDD, peer victimization in school students was prospectively associated with the development of BDD in which the symptoms appeared 12 months after incidents and also exacerbated low perceptions of peer acceptance [53]. With that, a conclusion can be made that experiences of bullying may play a causal role in BDD.

Moreover, the current results suggest that individuals who experienced physical and sexual assault in early life might be at a higher risk for developing BDD. Studies have shown that adults with BDD reported high levels of childhood maltreatment, with up to 79% of patients reporting abuse [54].

Furthermore, retrospective reported rates of abuse are elevated in people with BDD compared with healthy control. The BDD group reported more retrospective experiences of sexual and physical abuse in childhood or adolescence than did healthy people. This study provides preliminary evidence of the importance of examining abuse as a potential risk factor in the development of BDD [16].

Consistent with the other authors, emotional neglect was the most common form of perceived maltreatment in both males and females. Severity of self-reported abuse and neglect among females with BDD was higher than normal reported for women in health maintenance organization (HMO) sample. Consistent with previous research, females reported greater severity of perceived sexual abuse than males [55, 56]. Self-reported sexual abuse severity was the only type of maltreatment related to current BDD severity.

5.6 Parental styles

Parental communication styles with children also play a role in development of BDD. Individuals with BDD also report that their parents directly or indirectly gave more importance to attractiveness. Their parents are always commenting on various body parts of certain actors or actresses or characteristics of their friends as compared to themselves. It may also be that people with BDD are more prone to recall such information. Mothers' attitude toward their children's body shape will put their children at risk of BDD and eating disorders such as anorexia and bulimia when they communicate their preferred or ideal body shapes to their children through verbal remarks and the control of their child's food intake. Incidentally, this will shape a negative self-esteem and a sense of low self-worth to the child.

Although there is no current study to evaluate perceived family criticism of appearance, the researchers have conducted a pilot survey of BDD clients which indicates that familiar modeling and values are significant [57].

5.7 Society and media

Society and media also play an important role in the development of BDD. The media constantly reinforces the importance of appearance, while at the same time, creating unrealistic expectations about beauty. Although a correlation between the media and BDD seems reasonable, reports of BDD date back as far as the 1800s, prior to current media trends and the ideals it helps enforce. Furthermore, many standards of beauty and attractiveness are established before individuals are influenced by the media [58, 59].

Nowadays, media plays an important role in showing beautiful skinny female models and handsome male models with muscles. Children also are exposed to unrealistic body ideals, such as Barbie's impossibly thin, tall, curvy look with big busted shape or Ken's gigantic muscles. Barbie or Ken will be modeled after by children to look beautiful and charming. In extreme cases, this obsession to the models can lead to "Barbie doll syndrome", which individuals strive to shape a body like a Barbie doll. Constantly, watching perfect bodies can feed youth insecurities over attractiveness and weight. This is proven by a study where male and female adults show that being exposed to idealized bodies such as those in the media, increases dissatisfaction with one's own appearance. Research studies stated that our society's focus on appearance is a major cause of their BDD symptoms [10].

6. Cognitive behavioral therapy intervention of body dysmorphic disorder (BDD)

BDD can become increasingly worse with time if left untreated. Cognitive behavioral therapy (CBT) is the most practiced form of psychotherapy and has been integrated into highly structured package for the intervention of people suffering BDD.

Research has shown that CBT is an effective intervention in treating individuals with BDD [17, 34, 57, 60]. CBT can be conducted by individual session or group therapy session. Findings from the other researcher indicated that individual and group cognitive behavioral therapies are superior to waiting list for the treatment of BDD [61].

However, it is not yet clear how many sessions and at what frequency are most useful for the intervention. Psychosocial intervention studies for BDD have primarily focused on short term (7–30 sessions) of CBT [62]. Other researchers suggest 6 weeks of intervention with 30 sessions [63] and 12 sessions of 1 hour each [30]. The aim of the intervention is in improving the function and quality of life, in addition to alleviating symptoms of preoccupation with an imagined or slight defect in appearances and compulsive behavior [10, 17, 57].

CBT usually begins with psychoeducation explaining about BDD, followed by both cognitive and behavioral techniques. Cognitive strategies focus on identifying maladaptive beliefs, evaluating the accuracy of these beliefs, and helping the individual develop more realistic beliefs [31, 64]. The behavioral interventions typically consists of exposure and response prevention, which involve gradually confronting the individual with anxiety-provoking situations and asking him or her to stay in that situation without engaging in any rituals or avoidance behaviors until the anxiety decreases on its own. Often, the final session focuses on relapse prevention [63, 65].

6.1 Psychoeducation

Intervention for BDD typically begins with giving psychoeducation about the disorder. Psychoeducation refers to the process of providing education and information to those seeking for mental health services, and it is also provided to their family members. Therapists work collaboratively with the clients. The goal of psychoeducation is to help people with BDD to better understand with their mental health conditions.

Based on the assessment, the therapist focuses on educating the individual about BDD; features of BDD; body areas of concern; the CBT model of BDD; the differences between body image and appearance; BDD and cosmetic surgery; possible causes of BDD, including biological, sociocultural, and psychological factors; and also what treatments will be involved. This is important for their knowledge and view about BDD. Individuals with BDD also need to observe their behavior over time and situations to see what is working and where he or she needs improvement. Consequently, they can brainstorm and try out potential alternative behaviors.

It is important to explore factors in the client's current life that are serving to maintain body image concerns, including triggers for negative thoughts about their appearance, interpretations of their thoughts, emotional reactions, and maladaptive of coping strategies [17].

6.2 Cognitive restructuring

In cognitive restructuring techniques, the therapist challenges clients' distorted beliefs about their physical appearance by encouraging them to evaluate their beliefs in the light of evidence. Cognitive techniques included identifying their maladaptive thoughts, completing thought records, identifying cognitive errors, applying the downward arrow technique, and self-talk that leads up to rituals and blocks them from engaging in social activities like going out with groups of friends, going to parties, or dating. Therapists will introduce clients to common cognitive errors in BDD, for example, "This scar makes me very disgusting." Clients are then encouraged to monitor their appearance-based thoughts in and outside of the session and identify their cognitive errors, for example, "Why am I nervous about going to the party?" After the client has gained skills in identifying their maladaptive thoughts and cognitive errors, the therapist starts to evaluate thoughts with the clients [17, 66]. Cognitive restructuring entails evaluating maladaptive thoughts with Socratic questioning and identifying cognitive errors with the goal of developing more accurate and helpful beliefs [67].

Clients will be given homework for every session if necessary, and homework will be discussed in early sessions. For example, they were assigned to record the triggers, excessive thinking, and ritual behavior every time when the symptoms appeared. The aim of the thought record homework is to help client to step back from some of their thoughts and reflect on them. In addition, to help them monitor the negative thoughts that link to the repetitive behavior and help them to be aware of when the trigger comes up.

6.3 Exposure and ritual prevention (ERP)

A form of cognitive behavioral therapy intervention emphasizing exposure and response prevention has been shown to produce marked improvement in 50–80% of treated clients [68]. Exposure and response prevention is a process whereby the rituals are actively prevented and the clients are systematically and gradually exposed to their feared thoughts or situations [69].

Prior to beginning exposure and response prevention, the therapist and clients should review the BDD model to help identify their rituals such as excessive mirror checking, exchanging clothes, comparing themselves with other people, and repeated examining of the imaginary defect. In addition identify avoidance behaviors such as avoiding shopping malls, and discuss the role of rituals and avoidance in maintaining his or her symptoms.

Firstly, therapist and clients jointly develop a hierarchy of anxiety-provoking and avoided situations, such as clients often avoiding daily activities or activities that could reveal one's perceived flaws, including going to a party, going to work or class, or accepting social invitations. The hierarchy should include situations that would broaden a client's overall social experiences. For example, a client might be encouraged to go out with their friends twice per week instead of avoiding friends on days when he or she thought the nose looked really huge [17].

The first exposure should be mildly to moderately challenging, with a high likelihood for success. Exposure can be very challenging for clients; therefore, it is important for the therapist to provide a strong rationale for exposure, validate the client's anxiety while guiding him or her toward change, be challenging and encouraging, be patient and a cheerleader and quickly incorporate ritual prevention [17].

Meanwhile there are several types of strategies to eliminate ritual. First is using stimulus control which requires clients to manipulate their environment to avoid cues that triggers ritual. For example, if the client uses a tool like a mirror for their appearance ritual, the therapist should tell him or her to give it to someone else to keep it temporarily. Secondly, there are methods used to reduce time spent ritualizing. For example, if the client took 1 hour to check the mirror every day, the therapist asks him or her to reduce it by 30 minutes for the next day and then reduce to 25 minutes, reduce to 20 minutes, and reduce to 15 minutes every day and so forth until he or she spent only for a few minutes in checking himself or herself in the mirror. Clients are also encouraged to monitor the frequency and contexts in which rituals arise [17].

This technique will be more effective if clients are encouraged to use ritual prevention strategies during exposure exercises, for example, going to work (exposure) without makeup or delayed makeup (ritual prevention).

Doing homework is an essential ingredient of getting better. Homework is also given between sessions. It involves practicing skills that have been learned in therapy sessions. At various stages of the treatment, clients do exposure or behavioral experiments and ritual prevention as homework [10]. Therapists must always encourage clients to do their homework and give some credits if they did a good job.

6.4 Perceptual retraining

Individuals with BDD often have a complex relationship with mirrors and reflective surfaces. Clients may hesitate between getting stuck for hours in the mirror, grooming, or skin picking and actively avoiding seeing his or her reflection. Clients focus only on the body parts that are of concern and get very close to the mirror, which magnifies perceived imperfections and maintains maladaptive BDD beliefs and behaviors [17]. Clients also tend to engage in judgmental and emotionally charged self-talk.

Therefore, the goal of perceptual retraining is to develop a healthy relationship with mirrors, so clients do not check themselves excessively or avoid them and to view themselves more realistically [10]. The therapist helps to guide them in describing his or her whole body while standing at a conversational distance from the mirror.

Instead of judgmental language by clients, during perceptual (mirror) retraining, clients learn to describe themselves more objectively. The therapist encourages them to refrain from rituals or repetitive, such as zoning in on disliked areas or touching certain body parts. Perceptual retraining strategies can also be used to broaden client's attention in other situations in which the clients selectively attend to aspects of theirs and others' appearance. For example, while at work, clients are encouraged to practice attending to other things in their environment as opposed to his own or others' appearance [17].

6.5 Relapse prevention

Relapse prevention techniques may entail scheduling healthy activities to replace and distract from time spent on repetitive or ritual behaviors. The techniques provide clients with various types of treatment alternatives such as skills or activities that can be applied outside the therapy session. Clients and therapist will review which techniques were most helpful for the clients and how they can keep practicing them in the future after the termination of intervention. Clients also do other things, such as anticipating possible future stressors and how they can manage them by using CBT skills [10].

7. Challenges in treating BDD

BDD symptoms can be distressing and can interfere to some extent with living. Symptoms cause clinically significant distress or impairment in functioning. Milder BDD is more manageable. People with milder BDD may be productive, and some manage well despite their suffering [10]. People with mild symptoms are easier to engage in because they are aware of their illness.

BDD can also be more moderate in severity, and in some cases, it is extremely severe. When BDD is severe, it can destroy virtually every aspect of one's life. Some people will stop working and are stuck in their homes, sometimes for years, and some will drop out of work, high school, or college. Some even get into life-threatening accidents. Some suffer so intolerably that they attempt suicide, and some of them kill themselves [10].

Somehow, individuals with severe symptoms are more hard to engage in and refuse to go for treatment. Many of them are ashamed of their symptoms and are reluctant to reveal them to others [70]. Some individual with BDD are also depressed that it is difficult for them to get motivated to come for treatments. Most of them also do not believe how therapy interventions can help them to alleviate the negative appearance, beliefs, and ritual behavior [17]. Others believe that their situation is hopeless and nothing can be done to help them [17]. Therefore, they decided not to seek any psychological treatment and prefer to choose cosmetic surgery treatment. Some people with BDD also believe that they are normal and very healthy and, hence, do not seek any treatment. They think that their symptoms were not that bad. Moreover, people with BDD also tend to be very sensitive to rejection. Therefore, therapist must be careful to convey a sense of acceptance and concern without reinforcing their inaccurate beliefs about their appearance. In addition motivational strategies are very useful during the treatment sessions [17].

8. Conclusion

BDD is an issue of concern to many people struggling around the world. BDD is a mental illness associated with high morbidity and mortality, and early intervention is crucial for recovery to improve their life function. Treating BDD is very challenging for therapists, and CBT is a promised intervention for treating BDD [34, 60]. Therefore, research on psychotherapy for BDD is greatly needed. More research needs to be done to determine how well CBT works and which CBT techniques are most effective and whether other new techniques should be added for the effectiveness of the intervention. Research is also needed to find out for whom CBT works best and how to adapt it, specifically for adolescents and adults. On top of that, researchers, therapists, clinicians, and counselors are yielded to conduct more cross-cultural research in attempting to understand BDD culturally. Lastly, a study on a combination of CBT with pharmacological treatment is recommended.

Author details

Norzihan Ayub*, Patricia Joseph Kimong and Guan Teik Ee
Faculty of Psychology and Education, Universiti Malaysia Sabah, Sabah, Malaysia

*Address all correspondence to: norzihan@ums.edu.my

References

[1] Pop C. Self-esteem and body image perception in a sample of university students. Eurasian Journal of Educational Research. 2016;**64**:31-44. DOI: 10.14689/ejer. 2016.64.2

[2] Sarcu D, Adamson P. Psychology of the facelift patient. Facial Plastic Surgery. 2017;**33**(3):252-259. DOI: 10.1055/s-0037-1598071

[3] American Psychiatric Association. Diagnostic and Statistical Manual of Mental Disorder. 5 th ed. Washington, DC: American Psychiatric Publication; 2013

[4] Phillips KA, Menard W, Pagano M, Fay C, Stout RL. Delusional versus nondelusional body dysmorphic disorder: Clinical features and course of illness. Journal of Psychiatric Research. 2006;**40**(2):95-104. DOI: 10.1016/j.jpsychires.2005.08.005

[5] Phillips KA, Rogers J. Cognitive-behavioral therapy for youth with body dysmorphic disorder: Current status and future directions. Child and Adolescent Psychiatric Clinics of North America. 2011;**20**(2):287-304. DOI: 10.1016/j.chc.2011.01.004

[6] Sarwer DB, Crerand CE, Magee L. Body dysmorphic disorder in patients who seek appearance-enhancing medical treatments. Oral and Maxillofacial Surgery Clinics of North America. 2010;**22**(4):445-453. DOI: 10.1016/j.coms.2010.07.002

[7] Greenberg JL, Markowitz S, Petronko MR, Taylor CE, Wilhelm S, Wilson GT. Cognitive-behavioral therapy for adolescent body dysmorphic disorder. Cognitive and Behavioral Practice. 2010;**17**:248-258. DOI: 10.1016/j.cbpra.2010.02.002

[8] Phillips KA, Menard W, Fay C, Weisberg R. Demographic characteristics, phenomenology, comorbidity, and family history in 200 individuals with body dysmorphic disorder. Psychosomatics. 2005;**46**(4):317-325. DOI: 10.1176/appi.psy.46.4.317

[9] Buhlmann U, Etcoff NL, Wilhelm S. Facial attractiveness ratings and perfectionism in body dysmorphic disorder and obsessive-compulsive disorder. Journal of Anxiety Disorders. 2008;**22**(3):540-547. DOI: 10.1016/j.janxdis.2007.05.004

[10] Phillips KA. Understanding Body Dysmorphic Disorder: An Essential Guide. New York, NY, US: Oxford University Press; 2009

[11] Phillips KA, Diaz SF. Gender differences in body dysmorphic disorder. The Journal of Nervous and Mental Disease. 1997;**185**(9):570-577. DOI: 10.1097/00005053-199709000-00006

[12] Phillips KA, Wilhelm S, Koran LM, Didie ER, Fallon BA, Feusner J, et al. Body dysmorphic disorder: Some key issues for DSM-V. Depression and Anxiety. 2010;**27**(6):573-591. DOI: 10.1002/da.20709

[13] Veale D, Riley S. Mirror, mirror on the wall, who is the ugliest of them all? The psychopathology of mirror gazing in body dysmorphic disorder. Behaviour Research and Therapy. 2001;**39**(12):1381-1393. DOI: 10.1016/S0005-7967(00)00102-9

[14] Hadley SJ, Greenberg J, Hollander E. Diagnosing and treatment of body dysmorphic disorder in adolescents. Current Psychiatry Reports. 2002;**4**(2):108-113

[15] Phillips KA, Didie ER, Menard W, Pagano ME, Fay C, Weisberg RB. Clinical features of body

dysmorphic disorder in adolescents and adults. Psychiatry Research. 2006;**141**(3):305-314. DOI: 10.1016/j.psychres.2005.09.014

[16] Buhlmann U, Marques LM, Wilhelm S. Traumatic experiences in individuals with body dysmorphic disorder. The Journal of Nervous and Mental Disease. 2012;**200**(1):95-98. DOI: 10.1097/NMD.0b013e31823f6775

[17] Wilhelm S, Philips KA, Steketee G. A Treatment Manual : Cognitive Behavioral Therapy for Body Dysmorphic Disorder. New York: The Guilford Press; 2013

[18] Albertini RS, Phillips KA. Thirty-three cases of body dysmorphic disorder in children and adolescents. Journal of the American Academy of Child and Adolescent Psychiatry. 1999;**38**(4):453-459. DOI: 10.1097/00004583-199904000-00019

[19] Mancuso SG, Knoesen NP, Castle DJ. Delusional vs nondelusional body dysmorphic disorder. Comprehensive Psychiatry. 2010;**51**(2):177-182. DOI: 10.1016/j.comppsych.2009.05.001

[20] Phillips KA, Menard W, Faya C, Pagano ME. Psychosocial functioning and quality of life in body dysmorphic disorder. Comprehensive Psychiatry. 2005;**46**(4):254-260. DOI: 10.1016/j.comppsych.2004.10.004

[21] Gunstad J, Phillips KA. Axis I comorbidity in body dysmorphic disorder. Comprehensive Psychiatry. 2003;**44**(4):270-276. DOI: 10.1016/S0010440X(03)00088-9

[22] Phillips KA, Stein DJ, Rauch SL, Hollander E, Fallon BA, Barsky A, et al. Should an obsessive-compulsive spectrum grouping of disorders be included in DSM-V? Depression and Anxiety. 2010;**27**(6):528-555. DOI: 10.1002/da.20705

[23] Grant JE, Menard W, Pagano ME, Fay C, Phillips KA. Substance use disorders in individuals with body dysmorphic disorder. The Journal of Clinical Psychiatry. 2005;**66**(3):309-316

[24] Bjornsson AS, Didie ER, Phillips KA. Body dysmorphic disorder. Dialogues in Clinical Neuroscience. 2010;**12**(2):221-232

[25] Satel SL, McDougle CJ. Obsessions and compulsions with cocaine abuse [letter]. The American Journal of Psychiatry. 1991;**48**:947

[26] Phillips KA, Menard W. Suicidality in body dysmorphic disorder: A prospective study. The American Journal of Psychiatry. 2006;**163**(7):1280-1282. DOI: 10.1176/appi.ajp.163.7.1280

[27] Phillips KA. Body dysmorphic disorder: Recognizing and treating imagined ugliness. World Psychiatry. 2004;**3**(1):12-17

[28] Angelakis I, Gooding PA, Panagioti M. Suicidality in body dysmorphic disorder (BDD): A systematic review with meta-analysis. Clinical Psychology Review. 2016;**49**:55-66. DOI: 10.1016/j.cpr.2016.08.002

[29] Witte TK, Didie ER, Menard W, Phillips KA. The relationship between body dysmorphic disorder behaviors and the acquired capability for suicide. Suicide & Life-Threatening Behavior. 2012;**42**(3):318-331. DOI: 10.1111/j.1943-278X.2012.00093

[30] Veale D, Boocock A, Gournay K, Dryden W, Shah F, Willson R, et al. Body dysmorphic disorder: A survey of fifty cases. The British Journal of Psychiatry. 1996;**169**(2):196-220. DOI: 10.1192/bjp.169.2.196

[31] Wilhelm S, Neziroglu F. Cognitive theory of body dysmorphic disorder. In: Frost RO, Steketee G, editors. Cognitive Approaches to Obsessions and

Compulsions: Theory, Assessment, and Treatment. New York, NY: Pergamon; 2002. pp. 203-214. DOI: 10.1016/B978-0-08-043410-0.X5000-4

[32] Beck AT, Rush A, Shaw B, Emery G. Cognitive Therapy of Depression. New York: Guilford Press; 1979

[33] Deckersbach T, Otto MW, Savage CR, Baer L, Jenike MA. The relationship between semantic organization and memory in obsessive - compulsive disorder. Psychotherapy and Psychosomatics. 2000;**69**(2):101-107. DOI: 10.1159/000012373

[34] Veale D. Cognitive-behavioural therapy for body dysmorphic disorder. Advances in Psychiatric Treatment. 2001;7:125-132

[35] Feusner JD, Moody T, Hembacher E, Townsend J, McKinley M, Moller H, et al. Abnormalities of visual processing and frontostriatal systems in body dysmorphic disorder. Archives of General Psychiatry. 2010;**67**(2):197-205. DOI: 10.1001/archgenpsychiatry.2009.190

[36] Atmaca M, Bingol I, Aydin A, Yildirim H, Okur I, Yildirim MA, et al. Brain morphology of patients with body dysmorphic disorder. Journal of Affective Disorders. 2010;**123**(1-3):258-263. DOI: 10.1016/j.jad.2009.08.012

[37] Feusner JD, Townsend J, Bystritsky A, Bookheimer S. Visual information processing of faces in body dysmorphic disorder. Archives of General Psychiatry. 2007;**64**(12):1417-1425. DOI: 10.1001/archpsyc.64.12.1417

[38] Bienvenu O, Samuels J, Riddle M, Hoehn-Saric R, Liang K, Cullen B, et al. The relationship of obsessive-compulsive disorder to possible spectrum disorders: Results from a family study. Biological Psychiatry. 2000;**48**(4):287-293. DOI: 10.1016/S0006-3223(00)00831-3

[39] Monzani B, Rijsdijk F, Lervolino AC, Anson M, Cherkas L, Mataix-Cols D. Evidence for a genetic overlap between body dysmorphic concerns and obsessive-compulsive symptoms in an adult female community twin sample. American Journal of Medical Genetics. Part B, Neuropsychiatric Genetics. 2012;**159B**(4):376-382. DOI: 10.1002/ajmg.b.32040

[40] Monzani B, Rijsdijk F, Anson M, Lervolino AC, Cherkas L, Spector T, et al. A twin study of body dysmorphic concerns. Psychological Medicine. 2012;**42**(9):1949-1955. DOI: 10.1017/S0033291711002741

[41] Lopez-Sola C, Fontenelle LF, Alonso P, Cuadras D, Foley DL, Pantelis C, et al. Prevalence and heritability of obsessive compulsive spectrum and anxiety disorder symptoms: A survey of the Australian twin registry. American Journal of Medical Genetics. Part B, Neuropsychiatric Genetics. 2014;**165B**:314-325. DOI: 10.1002/ajmg.b.32233

[42] Yamada M, Kobashi K, Shigemoto T, et al. On dismorphophobia. The Bulletin of the Yamaguchi Medical School. 1978;**25**:47-54

[43] Turkson SN, Asamoah V. Body dysmorphic disorder in a Ghanaian male: Case report. East African Medical Journal. 1999;**76**(2):111-114

[44] Ung EK, Fones CS, Ang AW. Muscle dysmorphia in a young Chinese male. Annals Academy of Medicine Singapore. 2000;**29**(1):135-137

[45] Iwata Y, Suzuki K, Takei N, Toulopoulou T, Tsuchiya KJ, Matsumoto K, et al. Jiko-shisen-kyofu (fear of one's own glance), but not taijin-kyofusho (fear of interpersonal relations), is an east Asian culture-related specific syndrome. The Australian and New Zealand Journal of

Psychiatry. 2011;**45**(2):148-152. DOI: 10.3109/00048674.2010.534068

[46] Oh NR, An SY, Jeong MA. Relationship of BMI to body dysmorphic disorder among college students in Gangwon Province. Journal of the Korea Academia-Industrial Cooperation Society. 2013;**14**(7):3293-3300. DOI: 10.5762/KAIS.2013.14.7.3293

[47] Brito MJ, Nahas FX, Cordás TA, Gama MG, Sucupira ER, Ramos TD, et al. Prevalence of body dysmorphic disorder symptoms and body weight concerns in patients seeking abdominoplasty. Aesthetic Surgery Journal. 2016;**36**(3):324-332. DOI: 10.1093/asj/sjv213

[48] Jeremy GCG, Stephen L. Prevalence of body dysmorphic disorder and impact on subjective outcome amongst Singaporean rhinoplasty patients. Anaplastology. 2015;**4**:140. DOI: 10.4172/2161-1173.1000140

[49] Bohne A, Keuthen NJ, Wilhelm S, Deckersbach T, Jenike MA. Prevalence of symptoms of body dysmorphic disorder and its correlates: A cross-cultural comparison. Psychosomatics. 2002;**43**(6):486-490. DOI: 10.1176/appi.psy.43.6.486

[50] Bernstein IH, Lin TD, McClellan P. Cross-vs. within-racial judgments of attractiveness. Perception & Psychophysics. 1982;**32**(6):495-503. DOI: 10.3758/BF03204202

[51] Weingarden H, Curley EE, Renshaw KD, Wilhelm S. Patient-identified events implicated in the development of body dysmorphic disorder. Body Image. 2017;**21**:19-25. DOI: 10.1016/j.bodyim.2017.02.003

[52] Webb HJ, Zimmer-Gembeck MJ, Mastro S, Farrell LJ, Lavell CH. Young adolescents' body dysmorphic symptoms: Associations with same-and cross-sex peer teasing via appearance-based rejection sensitivity. Journal of Abnormal Child Psychology. 2015;**43**(6):1161-1173. DOI: 10.1007/s10802-014-9971-9

[53] Webb HJ, Zimmer-Gembeck MJ, Mastro S. Stress exposure and generation: A conjoint longitudinal model of body dysmorphic symptoms, peer acceptance, popularity, and victimization. Body Image. 2016;**18**:14-18. DOI: 10.1016/j.bodyim.2016.04.010

[54] Didie ER, Tortolani CC, Pope CG, Menard W, Fay C, Phillips KA. Childhood abuse and neglect in body dysmorphic disorder. Child Abuse & Neglect. 2006;**30**(10):1105-1115. DOI: 10.1016/j.chiabu.2006.03.007

[55] Silverman AB, Reinherz HZ, Giaconia RM. The long-term sequelae of child and adolescent abuse: A longitudinal community study. Child Abuse & Neglect. 1996;**20**(8):709-723. DOI: 10.1016/0145-2134(96)00059-2

[56] Walker JL, Carey PD, Mohr N, Stein DJ, Seedat S. Gender differences in the prevalence of childhood sexual abuse and in the development of pediatric PTSD. Archives of Women's Mental Health. 2002;**7**:111-121. DOI: 10.1007/s00737-003-0039-z

[57] Veale D, Neziroglu F. Body Dysmorphic Disorder. A Treatment Manual. Wiley-Blackwell. UK: John Wiley & Sons, Ltd; 2010

[58] Rhodes G. The evolutionary psychology of facial beauty. Annual Review of Psychology. 2006;**57**:199-226. DOI: 10.1146/annurev.psych.57.102904.190208

[59] Feusner JD, Bystritsky A, Hellemann G, Bookheimer S. Impaired identity recognition of faces with emotional expressions in body dysmorphic disorder. Psychiatry Research. 2010;**179**(3):318-323. DOI: 10.1016/j.psychres.2009.01.016

[60] Wilhelm S, Phillips KA, Didie E, Buhlmann U, Greenberg JL, Fama JM, et al. Modular cognitive-behavioral therapy for body dysmorphic disorder: Randomized controlled trial. Behavior Therapy. 2014;**45**(3):314-332. DOI: 10.1016/j.beth.2013.12.007

[61] Prazeres AM, Nascimento AL, Fontenelle LF. Cognitive-behavioral therapy for body dysmorphic disorder: A review of its efficacy. Neuropsychiatric Disease and Treatment. 2013;**9**:307-316. DOI: 10.2147/NDT.S41074

[62] Neziroglu F, Khemlani-Patel S. A review of cognitive and behavioral treatment for body dysmorphic disorder. CNS Spectrums. 2002;**7**(6):464-471. DOI: 10.1017/S1092852900017971

[63] McKay D, Todaro J, Neziroglu F, Campisi T, Moritz EK, Yaryura-Tobias JA. Body dysmorphic disorder: A preliminary evaluation of treatment and maintenance using exposure with response prevention. Behaviour Research and Therapy. 1997;**35**(1):67-70. DOI: 10.1016/S0005-7967(96)00082-4

[64] Geremia GM, Neziroglu F. Cognitive therapy in the treatment of body dysmorphic disorder. Clinical Psychology & Psychotherapy. 2001;**8**(4):243-251. DOI: 10.1002/cpp.284

[65] McKay D. Two-year follow-up of behavioral treatment and maintenance for body dysmorphic disorder. Behavior Modification. 1999;**23**(4):620-629. DOI: 10.1177/0145445599234006

[66] Veale D, Gournay K, Dryden W, Boocock A, Shah F, Willson R, et al. Body dysmorphic disorder. A cognitive behavioural model and pilot randomized controlled trial. Behaviour Research and Therapy. 1996;**34**(9):717-729

[67] Vashi NA. Beauty and Body Dysmorphic Disorder: A Clinician's Guide. New York: Springer; 2015. DOI: 10.1007/978-3-319-17867-7

[68] Sarwer DB, Gibbons LM, Crerand CE. Treating body dysmorphic disorder with cognitive-behaviour therapy. Psychiatric Annals. 2004;**34**:934-931

[69] Abramowitz JS, Taylor S, McKay D. Exposure-based treatment for obsessive compulsive disorder. In: Steketee G, editor. The Oxford Handbook of Obsessive Compulsive and Spectrum Disorders. New York, NY: Oxford University Press; 2012. pp. 322-364. DOI: 10.1093/oxfordhb/9780195376210.001.0001

[70] Grant JE, Kim SW, Crow SJ. Prevalence and clinical features of body dysmorphic disorder in adolescent and adult psychiatric inpatients. The Journal of Clinical Psychiatry. 2001;**62**:517-522

Chapter 5

Using Matching "Smarts" and Interest to Successfully Address Depression Caused by Existential Crisis

Michael Lamport Commons, Mansi Jitendra Shah and Mark Hansen Keffer

Abstract

This chapter outlines the background, nature, and explanations of existential crises. An unresolved existential crisis commonly causes depression. Crises occur in periods throughout the life cycle. They usually involve careers, relationships, or identity. The resolution often requires a development of a new stage of intellectual functioning, through which people can reflect on their interests and stage. The Existential Crisis Assessment measures severity of an existential crisis. A factor analysis showed the most important items in a person's existential crisis. My life, life in the universe, and relationships were the most important factors determining the severity of a person's existential crisis. The first solution is to match a person to a career. Another solution is to match one person to another. Three scales are used to match people to careers and partners: (1) decision-making measures how well a person addresses tasks of increasing difficulty; (2) perspective-taking predicts how well a person understands behavior of self and others; (3) core complexity interest scale identifies the reinforcement value of engaging. A further solution is that of cognitive behavioral therapy that can be used to both treat depression and offer training on social perspective-taking, a key ingredient to resolving one's crisis.

Keywords: model of hierarchical complexity, existential crisis, depression, anxiety, cognitive behavioral therapy

1. Introduction

Existential crises are seen as related more to periods in development rather than to stages of development. There is a main reason why existential crises are occurring more often and are increasingly difficult to resolve. The crisis is due to a constant increase in the number of choices that individuals face in modern day. For that reason, they are deserving of more attention.

An existential crisis occurs when an individual questions whether their life has meaning, purpose, or value. The conflict that occurs during this exploration can lead to anxiety and depression. It is important, therefore, to develop ways to help individuals alleviate these feelings and "resolve" their existential crisis. The main purpose of this paper is to discuss the several factors that influence how adults respond to an existential crisis and how a crisis can be successfully addressed. These conflicts serve as a stimulus for action while an individual searches for new sources of meaning in the hopes of resolving their crisis. This chapter turns to systematic findings from different areas within the psychology in order to analyze how and why changes in behavior take place during an existential crisis.

We unify the current work by extending notions of the existential crisis from something that happens during a "midlife crisis," to something that can happen at several periods in one's life: (a) the early teenage crisis [1], (b) the sophomore crisis [2], (c) the adult crisis [3], (d) the midlife crisis [4], and (e) the later-life crisis [1]. This discussion compares these crises in terms of features that are shared as well as those that are unique and also addresses possible influences.

In today's society, most people do not resolve their existential crises. Many people mishandle their crises and consequently do not resolve them. Such lack of resolution is mainly due to a lack of appreciation for the importance of resolving one's crises. Findings and discussions in this paper can serve as initial steps toward recognizing existential crises and their eventual resolutions.

2. The model of hierarchical complexity

The model of hierarchical complexity is a mathematical measurement theory [5, 6]. The model is a nonmentalistic, neo-Piagetian, and quantitative behavioral-developmental theory that analyzes the developmental difficulty of tasks. The model organizes task complexity. It proposes that tasks can be ordered in terms of their hierarchical complexity using an equally spaced unidimensional ordinal scale. It is used to predict the difficulty of behavioral tasks independent of domain and content.

The order of hierarchical complexity refers to the number of times that the coordinating actions must organize lower order actions. The hierarchical complexity of an action is determined by decomposing the action into the two or more simpler actions that make it up. This iterative process is done until the organization can only be carried out on a set of simple elements that are not built out of other actions. Actions at a higher order of hierarchical complexity can be described by several traits: (1) they are defined in terms of actions at the next lower order of hierarchical complexity; (2) organize and transform the lower-order actions; (3) produce organizations of lower-order actions that are new and not arbitrary, and cannot be accomplished by those lower-order actions alone.

Using the MHC, Commons and colleagues have shown that there are 17 OHCs [7]. The numbering of the orders and behavioral-developmental stages correspond with each other [8]. OHCs starting with the Preoperational Order 7, and continuing to the Paradigmatic Order 14, are relevant for adults. Because we estimate that 1.5% of individuals would be found who could successfully solve tasks at Order 13 (Metasystematic), and even fewer at Order 14 (Paradigmatic), most instruments constructed by those doing research in this area do not go beyond the metasystematic order. Only people performing at Concrete Stage 9 and above would be applying for employment.

3. Instruments

3.1 Existential crisis instrument

The existential crisis instrument was created to measure the extent to which someone is experiencing an existential crisis. This scale would be useful for counselors and therapists, so as to understand the severity of the crisis. The knowledge that one may be experiencing an existential crisis may push a person to resolve it by making changes in their life. The resolution of an existential crisis would likely mitigate anxiety and depression.

3.1.1 Method

Fifty participants filled out an online survey containing questions designed to assess the degree to which they feel that they are in an existential crisis. The questions in the existential crisis questionnaire are focused on three factors, those being (1) the meaning of life, (2) philosophy of living, and (3) relationships with partners.

3.1.2 Results

In the first factor, meaning of life, we have asked questions such as, "How often do you think about life's big question?" The highest factor loading was between 0.835 and 0.613. In the second factor, philosophy of living, we have asked questions such as "Does your work give your life a purpose?" The highest factor loading was between 0.780 and 0.514. In the third factor, relationships with partners, we have asked questions such as "How often do you change relationships?" The highest factor loading was between 0.728 and 0.668. Total percentage of the variance is 22.98%.

3.2 The decision-making instrument

The decision-making instrument (DMI) measures the complexity of information that an individual has considered in a decision-making process. Pascual-Leone referred to this as a measure of working memory [9, 10]. This assessment can be directly related to the task demands that certain jobs require of individuals as discussed later in (**Table 1**).

The DMI is based on a problem called the laundry instrument [8]. The laundry instrument is a causality task based upon Inhelder and Piaget's pendulum task [11]. The laundry instrument asked participants whether or not a piece of laundry would be clean after varying treatment. Participants are required to view a table depicting what has already happened (informational episodes) and then make predictions about what will happen in a new episode. Based on this method of construction, the DMI then consisted of tasks at the Preoperational Order 7, Primary Order 8, Concrete Order 9, Abstract Order 10, Formal Order 11, Systematic Order 12, Metasystematic Order 13, and Paradigmatic Order 14 in the MHC [7].

3.3 The perspective-taking instrument

The perspective-taking instrument measures an employee's ability to understand social situations, at least in terms of the notion of informed consent. Employees completing the perspective-taking instrument gauge the helpfulness and quality of guidance of varied hypothetical helpers. The perspective-taking instrument, like the DMI, is an online test. It asks participants to rate on a 1–6 scale the quality of six "helper" figures' arguments in support of their specific methods of providing assistance [12]. Each helper's argument corresponds to one of the six stages in the MHC, ranging from Primary Order 8 to Paradigmatic Order 14 (**Table 2**).

Stage	Decision-making
8-Primary	An individual's reasoning skills are low. At the primary stage, an individual can follow very clear and simple instructions but rely heavily on authority figures such as their managers to guide their actions and choices. The tasks they can handle must be simple and straightforward, such as stacking boxes, sweeping an area, and stocking a shelf. They can make simple logical deduction and can work unsupervised for only a moderately short period of time.
9-Concrete	An individual's reasoning skills are low. At the concrete stage, one must be given instructions but can make choices based on explicit guidelines. The tasks given can require various skills as long as guidelines are given. They can work unsupervised for a moderate amount of time.
10-Abstract	An individual's reasoning skills are average. At the abstract stage, one follows procedures and learns social normative ways of doing things. Therefore, they understand social norms and easily imitate what other people do. This individual uses abstract notions to make their decisions, e.g., best, coolest, never, anyone, or everyone. These notions are generally not completely accurate, but at the abstract stage, they are considered very important. When reasoning about a position, they use assertions that do not include fact or logic to justify their position. At this stage, one can work all day but need to be supervised a lot at first.
11-Formal	An individual's reasoning skills are average. At the formal stage, one can carry out instructions in a logical fashion of clearly stated policies. This individual is capable of making decisions based on empirical or logical evidence. They can work with one causal or predictive variable at a time. This translates to carrying out a single objective that is part of the greater whole, for example, solving one-dimensional problems, calculating interest rates, collecting marketing data, and writing reports that follow a format.
12-Systematic	An individual's developmental stage is high. At the systematic stage, one can be given instruction regarding goals without the need to dictate how the specific goals and objectives should be reached. They balance competing concerns and regulations and make judgments when there are multiple concerns and conflicting policies. They may supervise relatively large single units, such as one department. They understand unintended consequences and may adjust policies to deal with them. They calculate risk and understand its many sources and its costs and benefits. They write relatively complex programs. They do not need regular supervision. Performance of teams they supervise may be used as a measure of success.
13-Metasystematic	An individual's developmental stage is high. This manager constructs multivariate systems and matrices, for example, coordinating work between engineering and design departments. They work with the amount of information necessary to manage a team. They can put together a good team and orchestrate their work with marketing, accounting, and any other necessary teams.
14-Paradigmatic	An individual's behavioral-developmental stage is high (0.06% of population). These individuals are C-level managers and usually their own bosses. They are the innovators who institute the process, involve the stakeholders, and sell the solution. They tend to be long-term visionary thinkers regarding business models, objectives, opportunities, negotiations, external influences, and business direction in general. At this stage, they can develop operating mechanisms across multiple business lines to know and drive quarter-by-quarter performance in tune with long-term strategy.

Table 1.
Decision-making behaviors.

3.4 The core complexity interest scale

The fourth instrument used to job match is a new behavioral version of the interest test that is based on Holland's interest scale [13]. Our behavioral version is based on Holland's finding that people's "interests" have six different factors. These

Stage	Perspective-taking
8-Primary	Individuals appear immature in social settings and take the view of the manager even though it is possible for them to take their own view.
9-Concrete	Individuals lack social grace but can negotiate and bargain effectively with some guidance.
10-Abstract	Individuals understand social norms, easily imitate what other people do, have good manners, and are good at maintaining social harmony and pleasing others. They accept the company culture from a social norm's point of view and adopt professional standards as they see them modeled or as taught.
11-Formal	Individuals can revise social norms based on evidence or logical reasons. They understand social norms and can understand when a manager is needed to make a decision.
12-Systematic	Individuals balance competing concerns and regulations and make judgments when there are multiple concerns and conflicting policies. They may supervise relatively large single units, such as one department. They understand unintended consequences and may adjust policies to deal with them. They understand how to coordinate the different roles of people in the organization, particularly in one department, in a flexible manner to meet the short- and long-term needs. They can effectively deal with customers, employees, and the public.
13-Metasystematic	Individuals take the perspective of the various stakeholders including employees, managers, stockholders, and the public.
14-Paradigmatic	Individual sees that there are no perfect solutions but only partial ones. They involve all the stakeholders in negotiations to try to reach a consensus as to what to sacrifice. They ask each stakeholder to represent themselves realizing that no one else can do this. That is the way they come up with a way of dealing with conflicting claims and priorities.

Table 2.
The perspective-taking behaviors.

are as follows: realistic, investigative, artistic, social, enterprising, and conventional. The behavioral interest assessment interest test is much shorter than the Holland. The items are more clearly written in terms of task or activity preferences. It also uses a 6-point scale rather than a 2-point scale [14].

4. Cognitive behavioral therapy and depression

Aaron T. Beck's cognitive theory of depression proposes that persons susceptible to depression develop inaccurate core beliefs about themselves, others, and the world as a result of their learning histories. These beliefs can be dormant for extended periods of time and are activated by life events that carry specific meaning for that person. Core beliefs that render someone susceptible to depression are broadly categorized into beliefs about being unlovable, worthless, helpless, and incompetent. Cognitive theory also focuses on information processing deficits, selective attention, and memory biases toward the negative.

Cognitive behavioral therapy (CBT) aims to change our thought patterns, the beliefs we may or may not know we hold, and our attitudes and further helps us to more effectively strive toward our goals. In CBT, clients are taught cognitive and behavioral skills so they can develop more accurate/helpful beliefs and eventually become their own therapists. The beliefs that will be addressed in this chapter are about who the person is in terms of their "smarts" and their interests.

Cognitive behavioral therapy can help treat depression in multiple ways. Depression is an episode of sadness or apathy along with other symptoms that lasts at least two consecutive weeks and is severe enough to interrupt daily activities. Depression is not a weakness, but it should be treated. Negative thinking can affect a person's mood, sense of self, behavior, and even physical state, while CBT can help a person learn to recognize negative patterns of thought, evaluate their validity, and replace them with healthier ways of thinking. CBT can help treat depression by doing the following:

a. Utilizing cognitive restructuring and focusing on the immediate present.

b. Focusing on specific problems in individual or group sessions.

c. Being goal oriented.

d. Taking an educational approach to teach patients ways to cope.

e. Making sure patients take an active role in their learning, in sessions, and between sessions using homework assignments.

f. Employing multiple strategies such as role playing, imaging, guided discovery, and behavioral experiments.

g. CBT makes it possible to face conflicts and explore possibilities more directly.

CBT, combined with the abovementioned instruments, is a very effective way to help people through their existential crises and treat depression. We can get a score from the instruments which can allow us to determine what specifically is causing the depression, especially among an unresolved existential crisis. The instruments also reveal the severity of the existential crisis. With the help of all these scores, one treats the depression more successfully.

If someone is struggling with an existential crisis, a recommendation that may be made is to seek cognitive behavioral therapy. In therapy, a clinician may consider contextual circumstances. They may offer specific perspectives that may help the individual to resolve their crisis. The person might work with a guidance counselor or career counselor to see which careers, their interests, and smarts match. Through matching, an individual can attain results through taking all three of the previously mentioned matching instruments. These results may help to guide the individual.

It is important to note that the matching instruments do not consider contextual circumstances. These would include but not be limited to loss of loved one, end of a relationship, and loss of job. Therefore, it is necessary that the individual reconsiders their circumstances with regard to their results and how best to proceed in the choice-making which they will face in resolving their existential crisis. Indeed, matching is not designed to offer instructions for a person to follow exactly. It is only there to help guide a person better as they continue to introspect. Merely choosing the career that is best matched according to the three instruments does not guarantee a resolution to one's crisis.

5. The nature of existential crises

To live existentially is to question life's meaning: van Deurzen-Smith writes that "Existential thinking is an attempt to think about everyday human reality in order to make sense of it, and is probably as old as the human ability to reflect" [15]. From this, it can therefore be inferred that the ability to achieve consciousness elicits the ability to think existentially. Indeed, "it is the human psyche and his consciousness, which makes us capable of making meaning." The ability to think as an independent being not subject to ingrained evolutionary instincts allows for the consequential ability not only to make decisions for oneself but also to question one's existence through introspection. "Rooted in the work of early philosophers such as Sartre, Kierkegaard, Heidegger, and Nietzsche, existentialism came about as an approach to addressing the fundamental questions of man's existence".

These crises occur not as stages of development but as periods of one's life. The form and shape seem to be tied to age and role. The crises themselves arise at different ages and within different roles. If one crisis is experienced but not resolved, it does not mean that the crisis will last a lifetime. The crisis will likely diminish due to other factors that mask the lack of meaning within a person's life. Under such a mask, a person will not acknowledge their existential crisis until later in life when it will appear again. The mask can take the form of reinforcement. For example, in making a decision to pursue a career as bankers, these people might receive a lot of reinforcement from their job in the form of money, praise, etc. However, these people may also realize later in life, after these forms of reinforcement have worn off, that there is a lack of meaning in life which will be acknowledged through an existential crisis. In resolving their crisis, these people may decide to be a teacher and find true meaning in their life.

Furthermore, the resolution of a crisis earlier in life does not guarantee the lack of existential crises later. The resolution of an earlier crisis through which a person finds meaning does not guarantee that the source of meaning will remain constant in the person's life. A person's interests may change, and through a later existential crisis, they may realize the necessity of finding a new source of meaning. The experience of existential crises is natural to human development. It allows for a person to find new sources of meaning by which they can live their lives. Their occurrence cannot and should not be evaded.

In understanding the concept of an existential crisis, the logical inquiry would be to question why is it that only recently, existential crises have been garnering more attention from the society. This attention is the result of the increased difficulty of resolving one's existential crisis within the modern society.

In finding such *true meaning* within life, a person makes a choice out of the options that are presented to them. In this sense, the existential crisis acts as a fork in the road or rather a turning point through which a person is challenged with choosing the most meaningful course of action in their life. From this understanding, it can be said the expansion of the availability of choice in the society elicits an increased difficulty in finding the correct resolution to one's existential crisis. For this paper, *availability of choice* merely means the *existence* of choice within a society. The availability itself is not to be understood as being synonymous with the *accessibility* of those available choices. Accessibility here is concerned with a person's ability to access the available choices in the society. It is with such access that the person can then choose the choice which they believe to elicit the most meaning with their lives.

The availability of choice as an existence of choice within the society allows for a person to consider who they are and what will work for themselves. Making good choices will result in the most meaning and satisfaction within their lives. As Bigelow writes, "each man must accept responsibility for his own becoming." People must ensure that they are appropriately taking responsibility for their lives. Indeed, "an awareness of responsibility is in itself not enough to implement personal change." One must utilize that responsibility in order to gain access to the available choices that dominate the society while recognizing the necessary further steps needed to make the correct choice which will lead to meaningful changes in one's life.

The resulting anxiety of having to make such a choice is best understood using Barry Schwartz's law: "As the number of options increases, the costs, in time and effort, of gathering the information needed to make a good choice also increase."

Choice has always existed among the human society but only really started to dominate the society in the form of career choice during the Renaissance period during which urbanization took place. Such urbanization created more options within the scope of careers for wider populations. Indeed, "although nobles and the wealthy largely worked in the same occupations they had during the Middle Ages, increased urbanization expanded roles for women and the emerging middle class."

Due to the middle class being a small portion of the population during this time, it was still common for most sons to merely take over the businesses of their fathers, thereby involving little introspection. It was only during the industrial age that existential crises, as a consequence of further choice, began to occur more frequently. This expansion of choice is shown by the fact that "during the Industrial Revolution, due to the technological improvement, new jobs were created which lead to more job opportunities, thus emerged the middle classes."

This further availability of choice resulted in the pursuit by people to find a job through which they could experience the most meaning in their lives. In seeking such a job, these people would face an existential crisis in which they would reflect on all of the options available to them. It was a time of opportunity for people to find meaning that personally matched their individual lives. The commonality of sons merely taking over the businesses of their fathers was diminishing in place of further introspection performed by the growing middle class. Now, such availability of choice is inescapable. For example, high school and university, particularly in the USA, are structured so that people are constantly presented with different areas of study and interest, leading people into existential crises through which they must not only select a career but also discover who they are as an individual.

Such availability of choice within the US society increases the potential difficulty of the process by which an individual resolves their existential crises, due to the challenge of not only having to access the available choices in the society but also having to sift through all of the choices once they are accessed. The mere knowledge of there being an increased availability of choice in one's society makes that person's existential crisis more difficult especially if those choices are not readily accessible with ease.

Indeed, though everyone in the USA will face similar difficulty of shifting through the available choice, depending on the number of interests, as established by Schwartz's law, the route by which availability of choice is accessed is very much differentiated, usually by class, in terms of difficulty between different people [16]. Not everyone shares the same privilege of being able to make a choice without any struggle of attaining the means to make that choice. Such privilege increases the likelihood of finding the correct path that will elicit the most meaning in one's life due to the ease of accessing choice associated with that privilege.

Though such privileged, people may struggle as they attempt to make the correct choice. Their struggle will not compare to the additional struggle that a person may face in trying to gain access to an availability of choice. Bigelow references Kierkegaard, stating that "we encounter the true self in the involvement and agony of choice and in the pathos of commitment to our choice" [17]. It is only through the experience of that *agony of choice* that people can find the choices in their life that elicit the most meaning.

The additional struggle of gaining access to such agony is noticeable with regard to the differentiated accessibility of choice between the poor and the wealthy. This differentiation is explained by the fact that "class affects whether someone is going to be accepted into a particular kind of school, their likelihood of succeeding in that school, the kinds of jobs they have access to the kinds of friends they make." Each of these things determines and defines a person's privilege as related to his or her level of accessibility to the availability of choice within the USA.

Hence, little accessibility to choice is greatly significant in the scope of its limitation on the freedom of choice. Indeed, outside of luck and individual circumstances, in most cases, it is only through such access that a person can even have a chance at resolving their existential crisis.

These people seem to be caught in a viscous cycle, though which their limited accessibility to choice earlier in life systematically maintains their low socioeconomic status, thereby both maintaining their little accessibility to choice later in their life and extending the cycle to their children. It can be said that greater accessibility to choice correlates with higher likelihood of attaining wealth, and it is wealth that typically grants a person access to *choice.* Without choice, people will have little opportunity to find meaning in their life even though they have the freedom to do so. Indeed, the possibility to find meaning for such people is dramatically limited by diminished accessibility to choice.

The viscous cycle which limited accessibility to choice creates emphasizes the importance of true equal opportunity in the USA. This equal opportunity can only be achieved through a fair distribution of wealth across the USA, distribution that will provide opportunities for every American to lead a meaningful life. It is this misdistribution of wealth that is at the root of racism in the USA, as pointed out by Anderson: "True racism exists only when one group holds a disproportionate share of wealth and power over another group then uses those resources to marginalize, exploit, exclude and subordinate the weaker group" [18].

With the assumption of full accessibility to choice, in order to have a better understanding of the details of existential crises, it is important to consider the main aspects of each crisis. There are at least five existential crises that all revolve around the theme of choice: the early teenage crisis, the sophomore crisis, the adult crisis, the midlife crisis, and the later-life crisis.

5.1 The early teenage crisis

The early teenage crisis is concerned with, as suggested by Fitzgerald, one of the "greatest of life's tasks: the breaking away from the protection of others to find and define oneself" [19]. Through this breaking away, it is likely that a teenager will seek a form of individuality by changing their behaviors as well as their personalities. Through such redefinitions, teenagers change their behaviors as well as their personalities. These changes are a part of the developmental transition from childhood to adulthood developing organisms that must attain the necessary skills for independence. However, contrary to a common belief, hormones have been shown to have little effect on this developmental transition. Indeed, "gonadal hormones, have been shown to account for only a small amount of the variance in behavior during adolescence" [20]. The developmental transition and the attributed changes are rather linked to the teenager's learning of independence. This learning is reinforced by the levels of peer interaction which dominate the teenager's life: "During an average week during the academic year, adolescents have been reported to spend close to one-third of normal waking hours talking with peers, but only 8% of this time talking with adult. These outside-the-home relationships help to ease the transition toward independence from the family" [20].

The relationships themselves facilitate the behavioral change during adolescence. In understanding this, the reason for rebellious behavior becomes clear. "As noted peer interactions may also in some cases facilitate antisocial behavior, with peer conformity to antisocial behaviors including cheating, stealing, trespassing, and minor property destruction peaking in early- to mid-adolescence." What is important to note here is the idea of *conformity*. In seeking to find independence from one's parents, a teenager will likely conform to the behaviors that define their peer groups, typically one variable at a time. It is important to note that due to media, such conformity is not only influenced by peers but also by celebrities.

A celebrity's behavior and decisions will likely affect a teenager's choice of behavior and decisions. Indeed, a teenager will likely conform to the actions of the celebrity, therefore highlighting the importance of responsibility in celebrities whom teenagers idolize. For example, more and more in today's society, younger teenagers are sexualizing their clothing and appearance as part of their conformity to celebrities' self-presentations. It can therefore be said that depending on what is valued by either celebrities or peers, a teenager will likely conform to these values.

The reason for this conformity is more than mere consequence of peer pressure to *fit in* according to the highest-held values, whether those values be peer or celebrity related. The reason can be extended to the idea that as teenagers' developmentally transition, they displace their dependence on the behavioral values held by their parents and other adults with further dependence on those values held by one's peers or idolized celebrities for the sake of comfort. One article points this out in writing that "It is possible that this heightened conformity to peer pressure during early adolescence is a sign of a sort of emotional 'way station' between becoming emotionally autonomous from parents and becoming a genuinely autonomous person...the adolescent may become emotionally autonomous from parents before he or she is emotionally ready for this degree of independence and may turn to peers to fill this void."

Dependence on one's parents is all the teenager will have known before having their time dominated by peer relationships. Consequently, being dependent on one's peers will be the comfortable route of action for the teenager. However, after constantly changing their behaviors according to the current peer-held behavioral values, it is likely that teenagers will desire a form of independence defined by individuality. One study finds that "resistance to peer influence increases linearly over the course of adolescence, especially between ages 14 and 18." This resistance would be the result of pursuing independence. This pursuit is emblematic of a teenager experiencing their early teenage crisis in which they acknowledge their lack of independence and individuality.

Through this crisis, the teenager will gradually distance themselves from the broken amalgamation of peer values which used to define their identity. The teenager will be challenged by having to find the correct resolution to their crisis through which they can define their own personal values, independence, and individuality. Fitzgerald suggested "succumbing to the external pressures of conformity and meanings that are thrust upon one by objects or circumstances encountered in the environment it is solely up to the individual in order to create meaning and purpose in life" [19]. However, if such meaning and purpose is not created, the early teenage crisis will not be resolved, likely resulting in the teenager feeling lost in their identity. Such teenagers will likely experience depression, a side effect which is further discussed later.

Depression at this vulnerable age can have extreme consequences such as suicide. It is therefore very important that the early teenage crisis is resolved. The nature of the crisis and its resolution can be discussed developmentally in terms of resistance to peer pressure: "the growth of resistance to peer influence is a developmental phenomenon bounded by individuation from parents at its onset and by the development of a sense of identity at its conclusion." Indeed, achieving a sense of identity through independence is the goal of the early teenage crisis.

5.2 The sophomore crisis

This is the first existential crisis through which an individual begins to question the meaning of their life and how to find such meaning. It occurs during one's late teens or early 20s as evidenced by William Perry's "model for intellectual development in college students" [2]. The final stage of intellectual development, according to Perry, is *commitment*. It is the "integration of knowledge from other sources with personal experience and reflection; students make commitment to values that matter to them and learn to take responsibility for committed beliefs."

It is such commitment that is arguably required in order to resolve the sophomore crisis, commitment to one's personal sources of meaning. Furthermore, the sophomore crisis is related to the existential questions which Erikson poses: "Who am I? Who can I be?" These questions are the focus of a young adult's thoughts in relation to choice of career during the sophomore crisis [1]. Erikson writes that these questions occur from 12 to 18 years of age. However, this is likely an outdated range due to the recent influx of choices career-wise available to students caused by interconnectivity of the Internet age.

As Schwartz says, more choices will result in further anxiety over the difficulty of making the correct choice [16]. This difficulty requires an older age in order to sift through the many choices in career that are available to the young adult. The sophomore crisis is best understood as being rooted in anxiety over one's future and ability to optimally perform while delivering one's best intellectual capabilities. Such anxiety is typically the driving force behind wanting to resolve the sophomore crisis so as to establish one's identity as defined by a career.

If this crisis is recognized yet unresolved, the individual can find themselves feeling lost and panicked, feelings which eventually result in depression caused by the inability to find meaning within life. Indeed, the sophomore crisis is a major source of adolescent depression in today's society. It is important to note that some people may not suffer through this crisis if they have already decided for themselves what they want to do with the rest of their lives at an early age. These decisions, instead of being informed ones, are rather poorly grounded guesses which may turn out to be correct.

By *poorly grounded*, what is meant is that these guesses are typically based not on one's personal interest but rather on those of others. For example, young children may base their career choice on that of their parents or even their idols. In doing so, these children may grow older never considering their own personal interests, merely relying on essentially a *bet* that their guess was correct. In some cases, these bets turn out to be correct, and a person can fully avoid a sophomore crisis having already resolved for themselves what will elicit meaning in their lives.

However, if these guesses turn out to be wrong, which they often do, the person will face the sophomore crisis, likely with a heightened level of suffering. Such extended suffering would be the result of the individual's profound lack of introspection with regard to their own interests in potential careers before the sophomore crisis. It is therefore important not to solely rely on the guess which one might make as a child but rather explore one's identity so as to establish for oneself if that guess aligns with one's interests. Indeed, only through introspection and reflection over one's interests in potential careers can a person resolve their sophomore crisis, establishing for themselves the correct career path from which the most meaning in their life can be derived.

5.3 The adult crisis

This existential crisis occurs during a person's mid- to late 20s and is similar to the sophomore crisis in that it is concerned with making choices as to who you want to be. Indeed, it is an extension of the existential questions posed by Erikson ("Who am I? Who Can I be?"), being more complex in nature, dealing with things other than career path [1]. It challenges the person to decide for themselves who they want to be and who they can be. In resolving this crisis, a person usually becomes comfortable with who they are in all facets of their life, whether it has to do with the choice of religion, political party, familial dedication, level of introversion or extraversion, level of attachment to others, etc.

The list goes and is embodied by the choices by which a person defines themselves. In resolving the adult crisis, the idea is that a person becomes a fully formed, resolved, and individual adult who is comfortable with who they are as a member of the society. Along with resolving how one defines themselves, the adult crisis is concerned with becoming financially independent and performing adult roles, hence, the name, *adult crisis*. The crisis is the capstone of entering adulthood.

"The definition of adulthood that emerges from the GSS includes being financially independent, leaving home, completing school, and working full-time and further involves the acquisition of the skills and attitudes needed to perform adult roles." Interestingly, one study shows that this fulfillment of entering adulthood under this definition is achieved at a later age in today's society compared to the past generations: "The primary reason for the prolongation of early adulthood is that it takes much longer to get a full-time job that pays enough to support a family than it did in the past" [1].

This prolongation is the likely result of not only more choices in today's society but also the limited availability of jobs. As one article points out, "being a college graduate nowadays no longer offers the probability of a career." It used to be the case that in pursuing a college education, the security of a job would be mostly guaranteed. This is no longer the case and as a consequence, "In order to complete their education and begin work careers, young people now often linger in a state of 'semi-autonomy' during their 20s, combining support from their families with whatever they can make in the labor market and borrow."

The outcome of this *semiautonomy* is an inability to attain full autonomy through adulthood until much later on during one's late 20s, the peak of the adult crisis. Therefore, not only does a person need to become confident in the choices that define him or her as sources of meaning in their life through the resolution of their adult crisis, but they also need to have achieved adulthood. Not resolving this crisis can lead to feelings of disorientation and panic caused by a lack of confidence in personal identity. Ultimately, not knowing how to identify oneself in all aspects of life including your role as an adult will result in feelings of concern and depression.

5.4 The midlife crisis

This crisis in widely discussed in the media and is a household term, occurring during the early middle-age years, a variable age range. Wethington states that the midlife crisis is a term that "connotes personal turmoil and sudden changes in personal goals and lifestyle, brought about by the realization of aging, physical decline, or entrapment in unwelcome, restrictive roles" [3]. People often mistake this turmoil in life to be the result of high levels of stress. Indeed, though there is "expected stress" attributed with the midlife crisis, it is not the presence of stressors in life that causes the crisis. Indeed, there is a key difference between the midlife crisis and a "midlife stressor."

As one article points out, "common psychosocial stressors may have severe and long-standing physiological and psychological consequences." The stressor is best described as an independent variable which is viewed as stressing to the individual. The summation of these stressors is sometimes defined as a midlife crisis but is rather merely defined as the "overload stressors in midlife." In brief, many midlife stressors simply require the individual to resolve some of the stressors so as to relieve the overbearing stress that is dominating the individual's life.

A midlife crisis on the other hand is the result of reflection over life choices and the meaningfulness of those choices. As one article points out, "problems occur at the midlife transition when a person around the age of 40 perceives that personal growth has been stymied or thwarted. This distance between current achievement and aspirations arises from personal reflection at reaching a symbolic (or physical) marker of age." Within this marker of age, the individual is questioning the choices as markers of personal achievement (and meaning) that they have made in their life and whether or not they regret these choices [21].

The signs that reveal dissatisfaction with life choices during a mid-life crisis [21] usually revolve around career, partner, children, regrets over spent youthfulness, economic or social status, unaccomplished goals, and more. The length and struggle of the midlife crisis is therefore typically determined by whether or not earlier crises were resolved. Indeed, as one article reports, "the majority of self-perceived 'most important' turning points in life were reported as taking place in early adulthood, or even adolescence."

Insomuch as these turning points being able to elicit meaningfulness in one's life, if they were resolved, it would be logical to conclude that the struggle of a midlife crisis, which involves reflection over the meaningfulness of one's life, would be significantly lessened. Through the resolution of earlier crises, people will generally feel fulfilled by their life choices which elicit meaningfulness upon reflecting over their life during the midlife crisis. However, it is important to note that the resolution of earlier crises does not always imply that the sources of meaning will remain constant throughout a person's life.

Consequently, during a midlife crisis, an individual may recognize the necessity of finding other sources of meaning. In contrast, if earlier crises were not resolved, the person will certainly suffer through regret over their life choices and inability to have found meaning in their lives. In order to resolve this crisis, many will desperately try to correct their life choices in order to find meaning. Indeed, as found in one study, "many respondents connected the midlife crisis to life events such as job loss or forced unemployment, early retirement, extramarital affairs, divorce, separation, deaths of close friends or family members, and other major life crises, such as health problems."

Each of these events suggests or predicts a level of reflection over life and the meaning of one's personal life. Under this reflection, people will desire and attempt to find meaning in their life. However, many will fail, not able to deploy the energy and youthfulness that is required in order to make meaningful changes to their lives. The inability to find the desired source of meaning in one's life usually after years of attempting to do so will result in the *later-life crisis* through which a person will acknowledge the lack of meaning in their life and face depression and hopelessness.

5.5 The later-life crisis

The later-life crisis takes place toward a person's late 60s and is understood as a time of reflection. It is usually triggered by retirement, losing a job, illness, or death of peer or loved one all of which leads a person to reflect on their life choices and the meaningfulness of their life. This reflection is prompted by an awareness of the little time left in one's life. This crisis is further defined by Erikson's existential question: "Is it okay to have been me?" Within this question, Erikson writes that we engage in contemplation over whether or not we feel accomplished or satisfied with the meaningfulness of our lives [1].

People dealing with this crisis generally want to feel affirmed that they have led a meaningful life in which they have personally made a positive (or negative, depending on the sources of meaning) impact in the world. People who feel that they have led a meaningful life will typically and comfortably resolve this crisis and continue to lead a meaningful life. However, although having affirmed that they have led a meaningful life, some may not resolve this crisis and experience desperation as they try to make their lives even more meaningful before death. Such desperation can last until death and is usually experienced as an outlet of their fear of approaching death.

On the other hand, those who feel they have not found meaning in their lives will likely experience depression and hopelessness up until death. "Thirty percent of those who said they had suffered a crisis in their 60s said the long-term effect was totally negative." These negative effects are likely the embodiment of the depression and hopelessness which result from a lack of resolution within this crisis. People who experience these negative effects will believe themselves to have not led a meaningful life and, due to old age and little time left, will experience very little hope of correcting their life choices. The article states that in order to "avoid a late-life crisis in your 60s," a person should "maintain physical, financial and emotional health," "work longer," "use your time in a positive way," and "develop and maintain a strong support network."

Though it is true that doing each of these things will likely prevent an individual from experiencing a crisis in their 60s, it does not prevent the crisis from occurring entirely. They are better understood as avoidance methods which only dealt the crisis. Each of these actions elicits levels of reinforcement which will likely cloud one's existential thoughts through mere busyness. Therefore, though this reinforcement will delay an existential crisis, if a person has not led a meaningful life, their crisis will surely catch up with them.

Avoidance methods aside from one piece of advice that is helpful for potentially resolving the later-life crisis if a person has not found their life to be meaningful up to this point is found in Johns Hopkins Medicine: "Instead of lamenting what you never did, or what you've lost, Arbaje suggests thinking about this time as a chance to take on new challenges and embrace life in a new way" [22]. Indeed, this idea of embracing life in a new way raises the opportunity of making new life choices that align with the meaningfulness which one desires in life.

Through such embracement, the later-life crisis can potentially be resolved, though it is rare due to the difficulty caused by old age and a lack of energy. Indeed, "it is in accepting the reality of death, the fact that it will occur, that can give meaning and significance to living by emphasizing that our time is limited and therefore we must do what we value" [23].

However, such embracement of new potential sources of meaning is better deployed in pursuit of resolution of earlier crises such as the midlife crisis. Indeed, it is important to recognize that life is fleeting early on in one's life before it is too late to make the most of one's life and find meaning. The best method by which the later-life crisis can be resolved is through the resolution of one's earlier crises in life. Otherwise, there will certainly be negative effects from this crisis, elicited by an acknowledgment of a lack of meaning in one's life.

6. Conclusion

There are negative side effects to existential crises if they are not resolved, such as depression. If resolved, however, existential crises serve a great purpose in our lives, providing an opportunity to find meaning and purpose. The crises may push us through the anxiety we feel, to find the meaning. It would be appropriate to hypothesize that with more meaning and consequential satisfaction among the population, there would be less violence, more productivity, and more general tolerance among people.

Cognitive behavioral treatment will be more effective if the focus is more on the periods of life crisis and the stages of model of hierarchical complexity. A huge component of failure in treatment is due to lack of accurate matching of the instruments to an individual. Matching helps figure out at what stage an individual is at and helps us plan out an intervention treatment.

In future studies, we would like to match people to the causes of the crisis, for example, their career/job or their life partners, and resolve the crisis using the three suites of matching instrument.

Author details

Michael Lamport Commons[1*], Mansi Jitendra Shah[2] and Mark Hansen Keffer[3]

1 Harvard Medical School, MA, United States of America

2 Dare Institute, MA, United States of America

3 Georgetown University, DC, United States of America

*Address all correspondence to: commonsmlc@gmail.com

References

[1] Erikson EH. Identity and the Life Cycle. W. W. Norton & Company (Reissue ed.); New York: International Universities Press, Inc.; 1994

[2] Perry WG. Forms of Ethical and Intellectual Development in the College Years: A Scheme. 1st ed. Bureau of Study Counsel, Harvard University: Wiley; 1998

[3] Andrews M. The existential crisis. Behavioral Developmental Bulletin. 2016;**21**(1):104-109. DOI: 10.1037/bdb0000014

[4] Wethington E. Expecting stress: Americans and the midlife crisis. Motivation and Emotion. 2000;**24**: 85-102

[5] Krantz DH, Luce RD, Suppes P, Tversky A. Foundations of measurement. In: Additive and Polynomial Representations. Vol. I. New York, NY: Academic Press; 1971

[6] Luce RD, Tukey JW. Simultaneous conjoint measurement: A new scale type of fundamental measurement. Journal of Mathematical Psychology. 1964;**1**: 1-27

[7] Commons ML, Gane-McCalla R, Barker CD, Li EY. The model of hierarchical complexity as a measurement system. Behavioral Developmental Bulletin. 2014;**19**(3): 9-14

[8] Commons ML, Jiang TR. Introducing a new stage for the model of hierarchical complexity: A new stage for reflex conditioning. Behavioral Development Bulletin. 2014;**19**:1-8. DOI: 10.1037/h0100582

[9] Pascual-Leone J. Piaget as a pioneer of dialectical constructivism: Seeking dynamic processes for human science. In: Marti E, Rodriguez C, editors. After Piaget. Edison, NJ: Transaction Publishers; 2011. pp. 15-41

[10] Pascual-Leone J, Johnson J. Organismic causal models "from within" clarify developmental change and stages. In: Budwig N, Turiel E, Zelazo P, editors. New perspectives on human development. Cambridge, United Kingdom: Cambridge University Press; 2017. DOI: 10.1017/CBO9781316282755.006

[11] Inhelder B, Piaget J. The Growth of Logical Thinking from Childhood to Adolescence. New York, NY: Basic Books, Inc.; 1958

[12] Giri S. Cross-cultural homogeneity in social perspective taking: China and the United States. Behavioral Development Bulletin. 2016;**21**:176-183. DOI: 10.1037/bdb0000023

[13] Holland JL. Making Vocational Choices: A Theory of Vocational Personalities and Work Environments. 2nd ed. Englewood Cliffs, NJ: Prentice Hall; 1985

[14] Ramakrishnan S, Mei M, Giri S, Commons ML. Predicting success in academia using behavioral stage & Holland interest scores. In: Presented at the Society for Research in Adult Development; Salem, MA. 2016

[15] Van Deurzen E. Everyday Mysteries—Existential Dimensions of Psychotherapy. London, England: Routledge; 1997

[16] Schwartz B. The Paradox of Choice: Why More is Less. HarperCollins e-books; USA: Ecco Press; 2009

[17] Bigelow GE. A Primer of Existentialism. College English. 1961; **23**(3):171-178. DOI: 10.2307/373002

[18] Anderson C. PowerNomics, The National Plan to Empower Black America. 1st ed. Powernomics Corp of Amer; R R Bowker LLC publishing: The University of Michigan, USA; 2001

[19] Fitzgerald B. An existential view of adolescent development. Roslyn Heights. 2005;**40**(160):793-799

[20] Spear L. The adolescent brain and age-related behavioral manifestations. Neuroscience and Biobehavioral Reviews. 2000;**24**(4):417-463. DOI: 10.1016/s0149-7634(00)00014-2

[21] Emling S. 7 Signs You Might Be Facing A Midlife Crisis. 2013. Available from: http://www.huffingtonpost.com/2013/12/12/midlife-crisis_n_4419481.html [Retrieved 25 June 2017]

[22] Arbaje A. Healthy Mind: How to Cope with a Later-Life Crisis. n.d. Available from: http://www.hopkinsmedicine.org/health/healthy_aging/healthy_mind/how-to-cope-with-a-later-life-crisis [Retrieved 27 July 2017]

[23] Tillich. 1952. http://www.ehow.com/list_7484019_jobs-during-renaissance-period.html

Chapter 6

Neurosciences and Emotional Self-Regulation Applied to Mental Health Contexts

Prisla Ücker Calvetti, Fernanda de Vargas and Gabriel Gauer

Abstract

Mapping the self-regulation in the therapeutic process may be important to characterize the picture better, to contribute to the planning of the therapy and to select strategies for practical guidance of the patient, which will favor positive gains. It is important to know more and more the cognitive responses and behavioral characteristics of patients, such as associative learning, motivation and regulation of emotion, which may be linked to the genesis and maintenance of disease. We highlight self-regulation that is an executive function managed by the prefrontal cortex of the frontal lobe of the brain, essential to keep the individual active in the process to achieve their goals. It is a complex phenomenon that involves behavior (activation, monitoring, inhibition, preservation and adaptation), emotions and cognitive strategies to achieve desired goals. The neurosciences can contribute to the knowledge in emotional self-regulation in children and adolescents to health contexts in CBT.

Keywords: neurosciences, emotional self-regulation, health

1. Introduction

During the process of structuring the personality, there are many social and individual factors that can motivate or inhibit aggressive conduct. So it is necessary to consider there is a complex relationship between social risk factors psychological and biological, that is, the behavior is multidetermined by a set of variables [1]. In addition studies in the aforementioned areas are gaining space also in the field of law, since discoveries about brain development can contribute to the understanding of human behavior [2].

The advancement of neurosciences enabled the understanding that during adolescence there is an incomplete development of some brain regions [3], among these would be those responsible for behavioral control and impulsiveness [4]. In addition empirical research shows that experiences can produce alterations in the neural structure of the subjects, thus, it is reasonable to affirm that the cerebral cortex can be continuously remodeled from new experiences, from which comes the idea of brain plasticity in adolescence [5].

Therefore, studies in the field of neuroscience corroborate to understand the development of children and adolescents as regards the individual characteristics of adolescents in socio-educational measures. These findings may contribute to the proposed care programs in the implementation of the hospitalization measure can be more effective and coherent with the individualization of measures and the pedagogical character of the same. Appropriate interventions can enable the development of new cerebral connections and the change of perception about the crime, the fulfillment of the measure, the relationships established outside the institution among other aspects. In this way, it would be feasible to think that the integration of different variables, social and individual, could make socio-educational measures more effective. This chapter has the objective of shows the contributions neuroscience and emotional self-regulation in mental health contexts to cognitive behavioral therapy (CBT). For this, it is important to considerer the human development in the period from adolescence to adult life.

2. Adolescence: peculiar period of development

Puberty is a phenomenon that has always existed in the history of mankind, however the concept of adolescence,[1] as it is currently defined, began to be discussed only from the eighteenth century onwards. In this way, adolescence is correlated with many changes that have occurred at the cultural, social, economic and historical level in several civilizations [6].

In the eighteenth century, with the Enlightenment, a new movement of the society at that time, there is a redefinition of the social roles of women and children, as well as there is a new focus on family issues. The child is seen as the future of the family and the object of love of the parents, and with that there is a greater investment in the relationship between parents and children. At this moment the child is not seem merely as a miniature adult, but as a person, a subject of wills, rights [7] and peculiar characteristics. Still in the nineteenth century, adolescence becomes perceived as a critical moment of human development, which poses potential risks to the subject and also to society, and therefore becomes thematic studied among physicians and educators [8].

From this, it arises the need to specify the transformations arising in adolescence, physical and also behavioral modifications. The adolescence is defined by the psychological and social maturation process that accompanies or begins with puberty. On the other hand, it can be considered a biological phenomenon that produces physiological and morphological changes [9]. Thus, adolescence is characterized as the phase of the life cycle in which the personality is structured, and that there is emotional instability in the face of physical modifications that occur in body and the search for identity formation [10].

In addition to changes in the body, at 11, or 12 years old, some cognitive structures of the child also mature. The kid will develop the reasoning and logic needed to troubleshoot solutions. Piaget [11] called this period "formal operations". Among the biological changes of this period it can be emphasized the changes in the activities of different regions of the brain, which are part of the process of cerebral maturation [12]—childhood and adolescence seem to be essential phases in this process. Research shows that childhood experiences will exert significant influence on the development of behaviors in adulthood and that, environmental stimuli influence the development of different neural circuits in that period [13].

[1] The World Health Organization (WHO) separates adolescence in two phases, the first of 10–16 years of age and the second, from 16 to 20 years. Legislation Brasilian, according to the Statute Child and Adolescent Considers adolescent people between the ages of 12 and 18 years old.

2.1 Adolescence and development: neuropsychological aspects

It is thought that in adolescence there is neurocognitive immaturity, because there are some brain areas that are still in development. The situations lived during this period are also significant for the myelination of areas of the brain, mainly of prefrontal areas, responsible for rationalization, taking impulse control. In addition, recent findings show that this myelination may extend to the third decade of life. Previous longitudinal studies have already evidenced that the maturation process that depends on myelin could go up to the 21-year-old, according to the population studied.

In addition to an incomplete development in areas related to impulse control, there is also a higher intensity of impulsiveness in adolescents. With the use of functional magnetic resonance imaging, researchers observed that in a given task performed by the sample studied, referring to the gratification, the nucleus *accumbens*, a brain structure related to the reward system, showed a more pronounced activation than in adults who performed the same task. Thus, studies of this type corroborate the existence of exacerbated impulsiveness in adolescence [14].

It is during adolescence also, that the process of consolidation of different devices related to social cognition occurs, such as: the ability to interact with others based on the perception and recognition of emotions expressed by the face; the understanding of other people's mental states; and the regulation of behaviors in the face of an interpersonal situation [15]. These functions are of utmost importance in the face of understanding behavior. They are the ones that make it possible for subjects to interact, meet, perceive and relate to the world and the people around them. It is noteworthy that the interest in understanding the relationship established between the brain and the cognitive processes has increased in recent years [16].

Among the most researched cognitive processes currently, are the executive functions (EF) [17], complex mental functions responsible for the ability of the subject to engage in attitudes aimed at goals, that is, how this subject organizes and plans their actions in search of specific goals. Other skills related to executive functions are to create strategies, solve problems, monitor behavior, make decisions, abstract, reason, among others.

Moreover, the EF will allow the management of emotions and impulses, seeking a more appropriate response to the situations, what we can call autoregulation [18]. Considering that impulsivity can be classified as a poorly adapted response, without prior planning and associated with the desire for immediate satisfaction [19], the ability to resolve conflicting information and inhibit automatic replies when necessary, is understood as an indicator of the ability to direct future-oriented behavior [20]. Subjects who have decreased impulse control capacity can commit harmful acts to themselves and others [21]. Moreover, impulsiveness appears as a symptom of different psychiatric disorders, such as conduct disorder, personality disorder antisocial, personality disorder borderline, attention deficit and hyperactivity (ADHD), psychopathy, among others [22].

In view of this, the number of researches that have been focused on the neuropsychological assessment of impulsiveness and inhibitory control is increasing. Like this, the continuous performance tests (Go/No Go Task) have been presented as a promising task to evaluate mechanisms involved in the impulsive behaviors and self-regulation of the emission of motor responses [23]. This task is development in display (on computer) stimuli target (words, images, videos, and others) for the participants. These are instructed to press a computer key as quickly as possible (for the stimuli *act*) and do not perform any response in the presence of stimuli *don't act*, according to each task. From this, it is possible to observe three important aspects to evaluate the behavior: the omission in executing a response expected the realization of an undue response and the time each participant took to make the answers. The frequency of omission errors is often related to inattention in the execution of the task, while the frequency of commission errors is associated with impulsiveness and failure to inhibit a prepotent response. The reaction time for the responses, allows to identify the speed of the processing of the information [24].

So, it aims to evaluate the performance of children and adolescents in relation to the inhibitory component of executive functions, from Go/No Go tasks have been performed in different contexts. The study of Bilous, Small and Salles [25] with children presented as a result, to higher performance in the Go/No Go task in children in early school grades, being in agreement with other studies [26, 27]. That indicates the maturation of the cortical regions associated with executive functions with increasing age and with this, possibly the improvement in the performance of these tasks. With teenagers, this result is similar, [28] found differences statistically significant in the Go/No Go task performance according to the age range, demonstrating a chronological increase in the inhibitory control, in addition to finding differences in the performance between the participants gender (lower inhibitory control in females) and in private and public school students (better performance in private school students).

These results converge to the understanding that executive functions are related to different aspects of development and need to be evaluated taking into account different variables. Therefore, research in this field suggests that early interventions geared towards self-regulation are effective in promotion of executive functions skills [29, 30]. Activities such as, Yoga, mental training, aerobic exercises, among others, can provide ample benefits for the control of impulses, working memory and change of focus of attention, these skills, involved in the EF [31].

The Go/No go task has also been used to investigate the brain areas involved (activated) during the process of inhibiting responses, based on the use of neuroimaging techniques. An example of this is the study by Goya-Maldonado and collaborators [32] which found a positive correlation between the activation of areas of the ventrolateral prefrontal cortex and motor impulsiveness, during successful responses of inhibition a Go/No Go task. This study corroborates the interpretation that the prefrontal cortex is involved in the processes of planning, self-regulation of behavior and inhibitory responses.

The neurological bases of the EF are located in the prefrontal cortex, more specifically the region lateral and anterior cingulate gyrus [33]. It is noteworthy that the prefrontal cortex is not only involved in cognitive processes, because a region orbital frontal is related emotional aspects of the inhibitory control, so prefrontal lesions can also cause cognitive and emotional disturbances [34]. That is because the orbitofrontal cortex maintains connections with the limbic system, unit responsible for the emotions and by social behaviors. In addition, the frontal lobe comprises limbic structures, since the anterior portion of the cingulate plays an essential role in primary emotions, along with the amygdala [35].

In this way it is observed that the executive functions need the activity of several neural circuits, being correct to affirm that the whole brain participates in this process. However, the prefrontal cortex region is the last to develop, that is, to reach the maturational [36], therefore the EF takes longer to mature, and in adolescents this process is still under development. It is emphasized that the maturation of the executive functions occurs continuously, but there are outbreaks of development in certain ages of the individual, such as at 2, 6 and 8 years of age, lasting significantly until the end of adolescence and early adulthood [37].

When executive function changes occur, the syndrome, which is related to several cognitive and psychiatric disorders, may be related to neurological injuries or dysfunctions. In view of this context, there was an increase in research on executive functions, and about psychiatric and cognitive disorders related to dysfunctions of the same. However, as regards studies with children and adolescents in Brazil, most of the studies are about attention deficit hyperactivity disorder (ADHD) [38], autism, learning disabilities [39], and use of psychoactive substances [40], few national studies discuss the theme of executive function related to violence and the committing of crimes in adolescents.

However, international studies [41] evidence of low performance of executive functions, in neuropsychological measures, in individuals with psychiatric disorders that are associated with aggression, such as antisocial personality disorder, conduct disorder, bipolar disorder among others. In addition, several researches [42, 43] feature a significant relationship between cerebral dysfunctions and violent behavior, both in adults and adolescents, evidencing biological aspects as risk factors for this type of behavior.

In view of the above, it is observed that failures in the inhibition of antisocial behaviors are related to a less responsive brain circuit that does not fulfill its function of managing the behavior in a full way, based on social values established [44]. This occurs in both adults and adolescents, however, the phase of adolescence is peculiar, in the sense that the cortex prefrontal is the last structure to develop, which would explain some characteristics of this phase, such as, impulsiveness, difficulty in planning, limitation in braking the search for immediate pleasure and the fragile concern with the consequences of their actions.

In this sense, many studies have turned to the understanding of psychopathy and its development. Although criminal behavior is not an essential diagnostic criterion in this disorder, some central characteristics of psychopathy favor the involvement in anti-social behaviors [45]. Thus, even if psychopathy is a diagnosis that can only be performed after 18 years of age, many studies are performed with adolescents, seeking to identify possible neurocognitive dysfunctions and traces of the disorder that present some level of relationship with the picture in adulthood. One of the neurocognitive dysfunctions that has been investigated in children and adolescents, it concerns deficits in the processing of information about different types of emotional content, since such characteristics do not develop suddenly in adulthood, these deficits, traits and tendencies that can culminating in a psychopathic disorder can be observed already at early ages [46].

In this way, the besides studies conducted with adults, researches with children and adolescents have also been conducted in order to investigate deficits in the processing of certain emotions and have found of the convergent results with regard to the existence of these deficits in relation to the expression of fear, in children and adolescents with a tendency to psychopathy when compared to control groups [47–49]. Researchers have also found a relationship between the different facets of the psychopathy framework (affective facet and antisocial facet) and deficits in recognition of expressions, for example, the affective facet, related to emotional insensitivity was more associated with the deficits of fear recognition, while the antisocial facet was more associated with the attribution of rabies in neutral faces [50].

In adults, the results of studies show similar to those found in younger populations. Compared the performance in identifying negative emotions (anger, sadness and fear) expressed by the face, in criminal and non-criminal individuals with different levels of psychopathy, using the Go/No Go task. Individuals with "more severe" psychopathy presented worse performance than groups with "low psychopathy" in recognizing expressions of fear and sadness. These results reinforce the idea that psychopathy is related to the low ability to identify fear and sadness in facial expressions. Different studies have been converging on the diminished capacity of psychopaths in identifying certain facial expressions. Most of the findings suggest that there seems to be a deficiency in the processing emotional psychopaths [50].

Studies with neuroimaging also find similar results, since the limbic system, more specifically, the amygdala, are involved in this capacity [51].

These results may explain the “coolness” found in the psychopathic conditions, because a lesser capacity to respond adequately to other people’s emotions seems be at the root of different behaviors antisocial. Therefore, researches in this field can generate greater understanding about these deficiencies and contribute to the development of interventions of emotional recognition training, among others, in an early way, with the objective of generating greater effectiveness in treatment of adolescents with antisocial behaviors.

Finally, most studies and theories that sought to understand violence, involved almost in its entirety, social models and sociological, it is noteworthy that neuropsychology is also an area that can contribute in the knowledge criminal behavior. The attention on the anatomical base what involve these behaviors is important for the treatment of violence and the crimes present in our society [52].

In this sense, it is not about denying the importance of the environment in the formation of the subjects, but of recognizing that the social factors are relevant in the development the violent behavior can occur from an interaction with biological aspects. In addition, the experiences experienced in the environment contribute to biological changes that are related to the predisposition to violence.

Among these biological aspects one can think of genetic factors; hormonal factors; brain factors, both with regard to the structure and the functionality of the cerebrum; among other aspects. From this understanding, the subjects with violent or criminal behavior, can be considered as a “puzzle” biopsychosocial, that is, with biological psychological and social parts. Although several studies have already evidenced this relationship, it is still a challenge to understand how these pieces fit, or even, how biological processes relate to psychological and social processes.

Thus, it is important to consider the heterogeneity and subjectivity that are associated with the criminal and/or violent act, seeking to evaluate elements such as repentance, empathy, commotion, motivation, chronicity and severity of antisocial behavior. It is believed that these elements may present Indicative data on the need to consider. These aspects for the determination of interventions under the modality of cognitive behavioral therapy during socio and educational measures of hospitalization as well as other mental health contexts.

Author details

Prisla Ücker Calvetti[1*], Fernanda de Vargas[2] and Gabriel Gauer[3]

1 Federal University of Health Sciences of Porto Alegre—UFCSPA, Porto Alegre, Brazil

2 Federal University of Santa Maria—UFSM, Santa Maria, Brazil

3 Pontifical Catholic University of Rio Grande do Sul—PUCRS, Porto Alegre, Brazil

*Address all correspondence to: prisla.calvetti@gmail.com

References

[1] Gallo AE, Williams LCA. Adolescents in conflict with the law: A review of risk factors for infractional conduct. Psychology Theory and Practice. 2005;**7**(1):81-95

[2] Croat T, McCabe K. The brain and the law. Philosophical Transactions of the Royal Society of London. Series B, Biological Sciences. 2004;**29**(359):1727-1736

[3] Buchen L. Arrested development: Neuroscience shows that the adolescent brain is still developing. The question is whether that should influence the sentencing of juveniles. Nature. 2012;**484**:304-306

[4] Galvan A et al. Development of the accumbens relative to orbitofrontal cortex might underlie risk taking behavior in adolescents. The Journal of Neuroscience. 2006;**26**(25):6885-6892

[5] Schwartz JM, Begley S. The Mind & the Brain: Neuroplasticity and the Power of Mental Force. New York: HarperCollins; 2002

[6] Grossman E. Adolescence through the ages. Adolescence Latin American. 1998;**1**:68-74

[7] Osório LC. Teenager Today. Porto Alegre: Medical Arts; 1991

[8] Prates FC. Teen Violator. Curitiba: Juruá; 2002

[9] Piaget J. Six Psychology Studies. 24th ed. Rio de Janeiro: Forensic University; 2003

[10] Lebel C, Walker L, Leemans A, Phillips L, Beaulieu C. Microstructural maturation of the human brain from childhood to adulthood. NeuroImage. 2008;**40**(4):1044-1055

[11] Oliveira PA, Scivoletto S, Cunha PJ. Neuropsychological and neuroimaging associated with emotional stress in childhood and adolescence. Revista de Psiquiatria Clínica. 2010;**37**(6):271-279

[12] Beckman M. Crime, culpability, and the adolescent brain: This fall, the U.S. Supreme Court will consider whether capital crimes by teenagers under 18 should get the death sentence; the case for leniency is based in part on brain studies. Science. 2004;**305**:596-599

[13] Burnett S, Sebastian C, Kadosh KC, Blakemore SJ. The social brain in adolescence: Evidence from functional magnetic resonance imaging and behavioural studies. Neuroscience and Biobehavioral Reviews. 2011;**35**:1654-1664

[14] Haase VG, Salles JF, Miranda MC, Malloy-Dini L, Abreu N, Argollo N, et al. Neuropsychology as interdisciplinary science: Consensus of the Brazilian community of researchers/clinicians in neuropsychology. Magazine Neuropsychology Latin American. 2012;**4**(4):1-8

[15] Hamdan AC, Pereira APA. Neuropsychological assessment of executive functions: Methodological considerations. Psychology: Research and Review. 2002;**22**(3):386-393

[16] Barros PM, Hazin I. Evaluation of executive functions in childhood: Review of concepts and instruments. Psychological Research. 2013;**7**(1):13-22

[17] Tavares H, Alcarão G. Psycho-pathology of impulsiveness. In: Abreu CN, Strings TA, Tavares H, editors. Clinical Manual of Impulse Control Disorders. Artmed: Port Merry; 2008

[18] Blair C. Executive Functions in the Classroom. Encyclopedia on the Desen Development in Early

Childhood. 2013. Available from: http://www.enciclopedia-crianca.com/sites/default/files/textes-experts/pt-pt/2474/as-funcoes-executivas-na-sala-de-aula.pdf [Accessed: September of 2018]

[19] Del-Bem CM. Neurobiology of personality anti-social desorder. Revista de Psiquiatria Clínica. 2005;**32**(1):27-36

[20] Brandelero V, Toni PM. Test validity study Stroop of colors and words for inhibitory control. Psychology Argument. 2015;**33**(80):282-297

[21] Rossini JC, Macedo LBC, Teobaldo FP. Resolution of labyrinths and task act/not act in the assessment Atentiva. Psychology: Research and Review. 2015;**28**(4):796-803

[22] Bilous CF, Piccolo L, Salles JF. Performance of Children from 1st to 6th Grade in a Task of Executive Functions. Available from: https://www.lume.ufrgs.br/bitstream/handle/10183/45652/Poster_7194.pdf?sequence=2 [Accessed: August of 2018]

[23] Fuster JM. Frontal lobe and cognitive development. Journal of Neurocytology. 2002;**31**:373-385

[24] Miranda MC, Muszkat M. Neuropsychologistsa development. In: Andrade VM, Santos FH, Bueno OFA, editors. Neuropsychology Today. São Paulo: Medical Arts; 2004. pp. 211-224

[25] Willhelm AR. Evaluation of impulsiveness, inhibitory control and alcohol use in preadolescents and adolescents [master's thesis]. Porto Alegre: Psychology of the University Federal State of Rio Grande do Sul; 2015

[26] Diamond A, Barnett WS, Thomas J, Munro S. Preschool program improves cognitive control. Science. 2007;**318**(5855):1387-1388

[27] Raver CC, Jones SM, Li-Grining CP, Zhai F, Bub K, Pressler E. CSRP's impact on low-income pheschoolers' pre-academic skills: Self-regulation as a mediating mechanism. Child Development. 2011;**82**:362-378

[28] Blair C. Executive Functions in the Classroom. Encyclopedia on Early Childhood Development. 2013. Available from: http://www.enciclopedia-crianca.com/sites/default/files/textes-experts/pt-pt/2474/as-funcoes-executivas-na-sala-de-aula.pdf [Accessed: September of 2018]

[29] Goya-Maldonado R, Walther S, Simon J, Stippich C, Weisbrod M, Kaiser S. Motor impulsivity and the ventrolateral prefrontal cortex. Psychiatry Research: Neuroimaging. 2010;**183**:89-91

[30] Duncan J, Johnson R, Swales M, Frees C. Frontal lobe deficits after head injury: Unity and diversity of function. Cognitive Neuropsychology. 1997;**14**(5):713-741

[31] Fuster J. The prefrontal cortex—An update: Time is of the essence. Neuron. 2001;**30**:319-333

[32] Seruca TCM. Prefrontal cortex, executive functions and criminal behavior. PhD thesis in Psychology from the University Institute psychological, Social and life sciences—ISPA. Portugal, 2013

[33] Goldberg E. The Executive Brain. Rio de Janeiro: Imago; 2002

[34] Consenza RM, War LB. Neuroscience and Education: How the Brain Learns. Porto Alegre: Artmed; 2011

[35] Capovilla AGS, Assef ECS, Cozza HFP. Neuropsychological evaluation of executive functions and relation to attention and hyperactivity. Evaluation Psychological. 2007;**6**(1):51-60

[36] Gooch D, Snowling M, Hulme C. Time perception, phonological skills and executive function in children with dyslexia and/or ADHD symptoms. Journal of Child Psychology and Psychiatry, and Allied Disciplines. 2011;**52**(2):195-203

[37] Teixeira VPG. Changes in Executive Functions, Impulsiveness and Aggressiveness in Crack-Dependent Individuals. Alagoas: SayMaster's degree in psychology from University Federal de Alagoas; 2014

[38] Raine A, Buchsbaum M, Lacasse L. Brain abnormalities in murderes indicated by positron emission tomography. Biological Psychiatry. 1997;**42**:495-508

[39] Gomes CC, Almeida RMM. Psychopathy in men and women. Brazilian Archives of Psychology. 2010;**62**(1):13-21

[40] Jozef F, Silva JAR, Greenhalgh S, Leite MEL, Ferreira VH. Violent behavior and cerebral dysfunction: A study of homicides in Rio de Janeiro. Revista Brasileira Psychiatry. 2000;**22**(3):124-129

[41] Vasconcellos SJL. The Good, the Evil and the Sciences of the Mind: Of What Psychopaths Are Constituted. São Paulo: Icon; 2014

[42] Patrick CJ, Fowles DC, Krueger RF. Triarchic conceptualization of psychopathy: Developmental origins of disinhibition, boldness, and meanness. Development and Psychopathology. 2009;**21**(3):913-938

[43] Blair RJR. The cognitive neuroscience of psychopathy and implications for judgments of responsibility. Neuroethics. 2008;**1**:149-157

[44] Blair RJR, Coles M. Expression recognition and behavioral problems in early adolescence. Cognitive Development. 2000;**15**:421-434

[45] Blair RJR, Colledge E, Murray L, Mitchell DG. A selective impairment in the processing of sad and fearful expressions in children with psychopathic tendencies. Journal of Abnormal Child Psychology. 2001;**29**:491-498

[46] Stevens D, Charman T, Blair RJ. Recognition of emotion in facial expressions and vocal tones in children with psychopathic tendencies. Journal of Genetic Psychology. 2001;**162**:201-211

[47] Dadds MR, Perry Y, Hawes DJ, Merz S, Riddell AC, Haines DJ, et al. Attention to the eyes and fear-recognition deficits in child psychopathy. British Journal of Psychiatry. 2006;**189**:180-181

[48] Iria C, Barbosa F, Passion R. The identification of negative emotions through a go/No-go task: Comparative research in criminal and non-criminal psychopaths. European Psychologist. 2012;**17**(4):291-299

[49] Vasconcellos SJL, Salvador-Silva R, Gauer V, Gauer GCJ. Psychopathic traits in adolescents and recognition of emotion in facial expressions. Psychology: Research and Review. 2014;**27**(4):768-774

[50] Eisenbarth H, Alpers GW, Segrè D, Calogero A, Angrilli A. Perception and evaluation of emotional faces in women scoring high on psychopathy. Psychiatry Research. 2008;**159**(1-2):189-195

[51] Moul C, Killcross S, Dadds MR. A model of differential amygdala activation in psychopathy. Psychological Review. 2012;**119**(4):789-806

[52] Raine A. The Anatomy of Violence—The Biological Roots of Crime. Porto Alegre: Artmed; 2015